ASBESTOS CANCER:
ONE MAN'S EXPERIENCE

ASBESTOS CANCER:
ONE MAN'S EXPERIENCE

By Myrna J. Grove

Founded 1910
THE CHRISTOPHER PUBLISHING HOUSE
HANOVER, MASSACHUSETTS 02339

Library of Congress Catalog Number 93-74752

ISBN: 0-8158-0498-9

PRINTED IN THE UNITED STATES OF AMERICA

Dedication

I would like to dedicate this book to the members of my beloved family. I would also like to thank the following persons who were instrumental in encouraging the project: Kayta Dierks, Mabel Robrock, and Linda Sandstrom.

Contents

Chapter 1
Coping with Uncertainties

Members of my family are sitting on upholstered, cushioned chairs in the comfortable library lounge of the Olympic View Church of the Brethren in Seattle. Soft organ music from the sanctuary gently wafts its way through an open doorway. With brimming bookshelves along the walls, the carpeted room resembles a friendly living room. On the dark wood-paneled wall above our heads hangs a large color portrait of the founder of this congregation. Even though the white-haired, wise-looking man had died ten years beforehand, the presence of his portrait seems appropriate. Forty-six years earlier, he had had the ingenuity to first introduce my father to my mother.

Nearly half a century later, this cool June evening in 1989 could easily become another milestone in my father's life. This milestone does not involve a young man's first blush toward his future bride. Instead, it concerns the grown progeny of that previous union, who now gather at the request of their mature parents.

The current minister of the church, who spoke to us on the phone, now compassionately extends his arm in welcome. Then, he presents two older couples seated near him as being active members on the church's deacon board. My father rises and animatedly shakes their hands. Dad introduces each family member in turn, including my mother, my older brother and his wife, two teen-aged grandsons, and myself, his daughter. A casual get-acquainted conversation follows.

I lean back in my chair as I glance at my lanky, clean-cut nephews. Their questioning expressions convey innocence and concern. They have never attended an anointing service, and they listen with rapt interest to the exchanges. Dad mentions how the man in the portrait, the Reverend Dewey Rowe, had first suggested he meet my mother at a church gathering in northern Indiana. Rev. Rowe relished the role of matchmaker for youth in his unofficial pastoral duty. Dad admits that he was impressed with Miss Stombaugh immediately — so taken that he drove eighty miles to Ohio on weekends in his 1934 Master Chevrolet to court her. Rationing of gas made the trips a challenge in the early forties, but that didn't hamper his determined spirit. Dad says he collected gas coupons from others in order to make his weekly trips. When visiting, he would stay at the home of Mom's parents until 3:00 A.M. Saturday morning, and then drive home to Indiana in time to do his morning farm chores. As his grown daughter, I struggle to imagine my father so young and foolhardy.

In the church's lounge, the conversation shifts to illness and upcoming surgery which has prompted our meeting. One of the deacons tells us how his wife had once been seriously ill, but after a lengthy hospital stay, she eventually regained her health. His wife, seated beside him, slowly nods her head and relates how God's will can affect our lives and how the caring of others helps. I realize they are telling their experience to encourage us and to set a positive atmosphere for the service of anointing.

The Church of the Brethren anoints for three reasons. These include the forgiveness of sin, the strengthening of one's faith, and for healing and wholeness of mind, body, and spirit. The belief is that God grants these according to His grace.

Ministers frequently anoint church members who will undergo surgery or receive news of illness. Such services are directed at forgiveness of sin and peace of mind, as well as commitment to God's care. Usually, a minister is assisted by deacons of the church. Members of the family and the congregation may also participate in prayers for healing. My father, a deacon himself, had requested the service the day before his anticipated chest surgery.

The minister begins Dad's anointing by reading words of scripture which emphasize faith and instances of anointing in the books of Mark and Ecclesiastes. Concluding with James 5:13-16, he reads that we are to confess our sins to one another and pray for one another that we might be healed, because we believe that God wills our wholeness.

Then, the minister asks my father if he has anything in his life to confess which might keep him from receiving the full blessing of God. Lost in thought, my father tilts his head to one side, while he nervously rests a hand on each knee. A lump catches in my own throat as I consider the seriousness of the question. Dad hesitantly responds by saying, "I guess there are sins of omission. There are things I should have done and didn't."

With oil on his fingers, the minister then touches Dad's forehead three times while saying,

> Kedric, upon your confession of faith in the love and power of
> God, your willingness to commit your life completely to God in
> sickness or in health, and your desire to live your life for
> God's glory, you are now being anointed with oil in the name
> of the Lord, for the forgiveness of your sins, for the strength-
> ening of your faith, and for healing and wholeness, according
> to God's grace and wisdom.

Next, everyone encircles my father who is still seated. I rise, fal-
teringly, feeling my knees weaken. The minister instructs us to
place our hands on Dad's shoulders and head. I gaze downward,
reaching for his right shoulder as my left hand clutches a Kleenex.
Sensing my struggle, the deaconess next to me calmly lays her
hand over mine.

During prayer, we are asked if anyone wants to speak. I can
barely stand, let alone utter any thoughts. My eyes unexpectedly
fill with tears. My father has never been ill or spent a day in the
hospital in his life. I am unused to seeing him in this vulnerable
state. What would the next day of surgery bring? How would he
tolerate it? What was God preparing us for? Fears and uncertainties swim around in my head.

My sister-in-law Mary expresses how much we love my father
and how vital he is in our lives. In a cracking voice, my brother
Dean shares similar sentiments. My nephew Derek, standing
behind me, puts a firm hand on my shoulder. His action holds me
up, as I sob audibly. Words choke in my throat. The deacons and
minister add messages of healing before closing. I wish I had been
able to speak. I am grateful to those who did.

Dad smiles as we step back from him. "I feel better now," he
says. "I'm ready for what is to come."

Chapter 2
Of Undetermined Origin

The previous four months had started simply enough. In January of 1989, my mother encouraged Dad to get a routine physical. Mother was scheduling her periodic checkup, and she thought Dad should do the same. At the time, he suffered no known physical symptoms and, in some ways, had never felt better.

In his ninth year of retirement from the Central Foundry Division of General Motors, Dad remained quite active, both physically and mentally. He jogged several times a week and watched his cholesterol intake when eating. His tall, strong frame had never been overweight.

My parents made their appointments at the local medical center in Bryan, Ohio, a light industrial town located in northwest Ohio. I paid slight attention, assuming they could handle the arrangements.

Both Dad and Mom were near seventy years of age, and so far, had few physical problems. Mom's limp from a childhood bout with polio slowed her walking pace, and she took medication for high blood pressure. Dad usually even refused to take aspirin, and he prided himself on his hardy, physical endurance.

I expected my parents to survive for a long time. My maternal grandfather had died only five years before, at age ninety-four. Mom's side of the family was noted for long life spans, and Dad had been nearly fifty when his parents died. In my calculations, Mom's longevity and Dad's physical hardiness would sustain them for another twenty years. Then, when my generation had acquired sufficient wisdom and gray hair, the torch would be passed. Isn't that how it's supposed to work?

For now, my parents actively engaged in living. They were planning more trips. They often participated in retirement meetings, both for the county teachers and for my father's unit of the United Auto Workers. Mother was president of Williams County

Community Concerts. Dad mowed the lawn at their country home, designed and built bookcases, and puttered with family cars. And both of them were involved in numerous church programs.

In fact, Dad could win a Bible quiz handily. He had taught Sunday School for many years. Previously, he taught the adult class called the Helping Hands, which included my maternal grandparents. When that group advanced to its heavenly home, Dad adopted another class of senior citizens known as the Golden Rule. He kept a Bible on the night stand by his bed. The interaction of Biblical characters fascinated him as he repeatedly read his favorite stories.

As a young man, Dad had been elected a church deacon by the Pleasant Valley Church of the Brethren near Middlebury, Indiana. In the denomination, deacons are chosen for life terms by the church membership to give spiritual guidance. After my father's marriage and move to northern Ohio, his deacon responsibilities transferred to his new congregation.

In Ohio, Dad was elected as a member of the church board's witness commission. He faithfully kept minutes of the proceedings. His most recent church post was as church treasurer, a job he handled meticulously.

Thus, even at the age of seventy-one, life for my father was an active, involved effort. He scheduled a routine physical to please my mother. Mom had received good reports on her tests, and Dad thought his would go as well. His doctor gave him a general checkup and blood tests one day and a chest X-ray the next.

A series of medical appointments took root even then. The day after the X-ray, the nurse called and asked Dad to return to the medical center. The doctor had found an unusual dark spot on his right lung. This time, Dad should report for a CAT scan of his chest. CAT stands for Computerized Axial Tomography, which is actually a more detailed X-ray.

A day after the CAT scan, Dad met with his doctor to discuss the results. The CAT scan revealed a "pleural based density just to the right of the midline at the level of the aortic arch." The outer margin of this was somewhat irregular. The doctor thought this might be nothing more than pleural thickening, although he felt a needle biopsy would help rule out a tumor. There were smaller pleural based densities on the right back. Pleural refers to the lining, or membrane, that encases the lungs. The doctor recommended a biopsy of the right lung, and he referred Dad to a local surgeon.

The surgeon explained that he would remove a small piece of

tissue to examine under a microscope, and he arranged the biopsy for the following day. Dad was not unusually alarmed. If anything serious was wrong, why would he feel this good? However, Mom began reporting these daily doctor visits to my brothers and me, especially my older brother who was a physician in the Seattle, Washington, area.

A week later, the biopsy results were back. The specimen examined was two tissue fragments measuring one-tenth centimeter in size. Microscopy study showed cells from the respiratory lining which had slightly enlarged nuclei. No cancer cells were visible. My father was advised to return in three months, and the doctor would study the lung area to see if further growth had developed.

It had been a long week. The slight fear that there was something wrong gave way to tremendous relief that life would go on as usual. Dad would return for a second chest CAT scan in May. Meanwhile, he could resume his daily plans and perhaps plant some spring flowers. A week later, during his heart stress test, he performed skillfully on the treadmill.

Outwardly, Dad showed no signs of concern about his physical condition. In the next three months, he rarely brought it up in conversation. He did write to his sister in Indiana and his brother-in-law in Texas that an unusual dark spot had been found on his lung. He added that doctors couldn't identify the atypical cells, and they would re-examine them later.

Dad continued his usual activities in the spring of 1989. He bought new jogging sneakers. He started his yard work routine. He chaired deacon meetings and attended church services. He drove my mother to her district church board meeting in eastern Ohio. And with Mom, he attended her fiftieth college class reunion at Manchester College in Indiana. During the spring months of new life, Dad experienced a reprieve from future inevitable events.

Chapter 3
Finding Roots

Our first American ancestors were Swiss Mennonites who had fled from the canton of Zurich to the Palatinate area of Germany and immigrated to Philadelphia in the 1700s. Graf was traditionally a Mennonite name in that area of Europe, and the spelling further evolved from Groff to Grove in America. An early ancestor, John Groff, known as "Swamp John," was born in 1715 and died in 1777 near Strasburg, Pennsylvania. He married Catherine Herr who was born in 1727 in New Providence, Pennsylvania. Catherine's grandfather was the Rev. Hans Herr, a Mennonite minister, who had contracted with William Penn for 10,000 acres of land in what later became Lancaster County, moving there in 1710 with his extended family.

In Europe, the Anabaptist groups had been persecuted because of their opposition to the state church. The term Anabaptist started as a nickname meaning rebaptizer because the Anabaptist groups rejected infant baptism. Other beliefs included emphasis on obedience to the New Testament, separation of church and state, nonparticipation in military service, and imitation of Jesus' life and character within a community.

The Mennonites in Lancaster County were neighbors of other Anabaptist groups who had come to Pennsylvania for freedom of religion. After the Civil War, my ancestors joined the Church of the Brethren. This denomination was also inspired by the Pietist-Anabaptist movement, and founded in Germany in 1708. Members immigrated to Germantown, Pennsylvania, around 1720. The church shares many beliefs in common with the Mennonites, Amish, and Quakers, and all four are considered historic peace churches.

Prior to the Revolutionary War, Pennsylvania Germans began migrating south to the Shenandoah Valley of Virginia seeking better land and better economic conditions. By the 1790s, the move-

9

ment of German-speaking settlers reached such significant numbers that the German language was the predominant tongue. Martin Groff and Benjamin Groff, two sons of Swamp John, joined this migration.

My great-great-great-great-grandfather, Martin Groff, and his wife Anna Kendig, moved in 1792 from Pennsylvania to Augusta County, Virginia, part of the plush valley. The Martin Groffs raised twelve children, including my thrice great-grandfather, Abraham Grove, whose name acquired the English spelling. During the "Roots" era of the seventies, I had often wondered about the Groves since I seldom encountered our surname in northwest Ohio. I found these early Grove graves on the edge of the Martin Groff farm near Hermitage and in the Mount Vernon Church of the Brethren cemetery south of Waynesboro, Virginia.

The Abraham Grove family settled on what had been Stuart land southwest of Waynesboro, known as the South River region. According to my great-grandfather's will, the Groves owned four farms southwest of town and two grazing farms in the mountains, one in Augusta County and one in Albermarle County. The original homestead, built in 1804, was an L-shaped, two-story brick house in a country neo-classical style. No longer standing, the homestead's location is now the site of the P. Buckley Moss Museum. Moss is an internationally acclaimed artist of Amish and Mennonite scenes.

My great-great-grandfather's name was John Grove. He is said to have paid someone to fight for him in the Civil War, a practice by some pacifists. After John, three more generations of Groves were born on the rich farmland of the upper Shenandoah Valley, including my grandfather Alvin Grove. Alvin was the second oldest of five surviving children of Charles and Cora Flory Grove. His mother died at age 37 when Alvin was an impressionable thirteen. Soon, his father Charles married a young bride who bore four more children. Alvin became the first among his siblings to leave Virginia.

Alvin's exit was an unplanned event. Along with his older brothers, he worked on his father's farms. At the age of seventeen, Alvin was forbidden by his father to attend a school dance. His father said that if Alvin went to the dance, he needn't bother to come home. Well, Alvin stubbornly enjoyed the dance, and then departed the same night for his Uncle Will's farm in Iowa. He was gone for about a year while he worked on his uncle's farm. Then, he returned briefly to Virginia and convinced his older brother Earl to accompany him to Iowa. Thus, the two oldest Grove brothers moved to the North where both of them met their future wives.

My paternal grandmother, Kathryn Edna Everhock, had traveled from Indiana by train to visit her favorite Aunt Annie Coffman near Keswick, Iowa. During her stay, she met the wandering Virginian, Alvin Miller Grove. In 1913, they were married in her hometown of Millersburg, Indiana, when Alvin was twenty and Kathryn was twenty-two.

With his new bride, Alvin attempted once more to return to his native Virginia. Alvin and Kathryn rented a farm from his father where their first son Ronald was born in 1915.

But when my father Kedric was born in 1917, Alvin and Kathryn had already moved back to northern Indiana. Dad used to say he was the second son of the second son. Later, Dad could include his own second son who has a second son.

Wanderlust had still not been satisfied when the Alvin Grove family, with baby Carolyn now added, moved south to Jacksonville, Florida, in 1927-28. Alvin needed work, and Kathryn thought the warm winters would aid her health. Alvin spent the winter picking oranges. Because the work was seasonal, the family moved to Long Island, New York, in between moves back to Florida. Dad once told how painfully shy he had been when attending the fourth grade in Jacksonville. His brother Ronald had protected him from the bullies who teased them for being "Northerners."

Next, in 1929, Alvin became a sharecropper on the farm of his wife's brother near Millersburg, Indiana. My father Kedric, who had been taken in and out of schools, started high school in Millersburg. By his junior year, the family uprooted again to a rented farm near Bristol, Indiana. Dad hated switching schools yet another time, and he threatened to quit. After witnessing his mother's tears, he reluctantly enrolled and later graduated from Bristol High School in 1935. With his friendly manner, Dad had easily made new friends. His favorite subject in high school was drawing, and he also liked to read. In later years, Dad attended the high school reunions at both Millersburg and Bristol. He reported that his old high school in Bristol has now been converted into the Elkhart County Museum, where photos of former graduating classes hang in the hallways.

During the Depression, Dad was not inclined to go to college. His parents neither encouraged nor could afford to send him, and Dad practiced his mechanical ability and his skill with animals instead of pursuing academics. To earn money, his father and he bought calves to raise and sell.

In the spring of 1937, the Grove family traveled to Idaho. They rented a home near Nampa, where they picked potatoes, onions, and apples. But by August, they were enroute to Iowa. And by November, the family had again settled in Indiana, where son Ronald bought a two-story house for them near Middlebury.

Near this time, Dad's mother Kathryn started nurses' training by correspondence from the Chicago School of Nursing. She later worked as an aide at Elkhart Hospital. As a licensed practical nurse, she also provided live-in health care for area patients. Alvin worked as a night watchman at Caswell Runyan Factory, a plywood veneer manufacturer in Goshen.

As a young man, Dad decided to follow a common stage for youthful adventurers and go to Florida. He purchased a trailer, which was really half-tent, and settled in Winter Park. Later, he sold his trailer and rented a cottage. When spring arrived, he returned to Indiana and worked on a farm near his parents.

Suddenly, the government was calling men to service in World War II. Dad registered, passed his physical, but was not drafted. By now, he was twenty-five years old, and most of the draftees were in the 18-22 year old range. Dad received a deferment to stay home and farm. In addition, his Church of the Brethren beliefs upheld peaceful resistance to the war.

Despite being uprooted frequently during his childhood, Dad held no ill will toward his parents. Even though Alvin spoke with a raucous voice and was rather stiff and stern-faced, the neighbors considered the Grove family to be quiet and peaceful.

They had survived the Depression by moving around, and had kept their strong religious faith. Although they did not own a large collection of books, both of Dad's parents read voraciously. His mother collected poetry books and published some of her own pieces.

Soon after his return from Florida, Dad met my mother while both were attending services held at his church near Middlebury, Indiana. Her Ohio pastor had filled the role of matchmaker. A year later, my parents were married on Valentine's Day of 1943, at the Lick Creek Church of the Brethren in northwest Ohio. From then on, Dad claimed firm roots in one location.

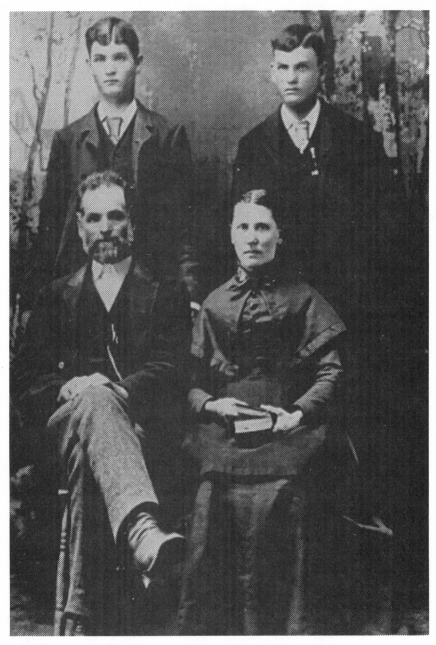

John and Sarah Grove family of Waynesboro, Virginia, circa 1880s, with sons William and Charles Jacob, my father's grandfather.

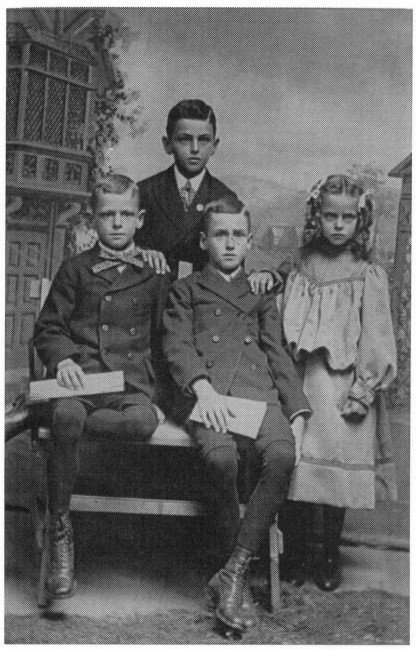

The first four children of Charles (C.J.) and Cora Flory Grove, Waynesboro, Virginia. From left, Raymond, Earl (standing), Alvin, my Dad's father, and Edith.

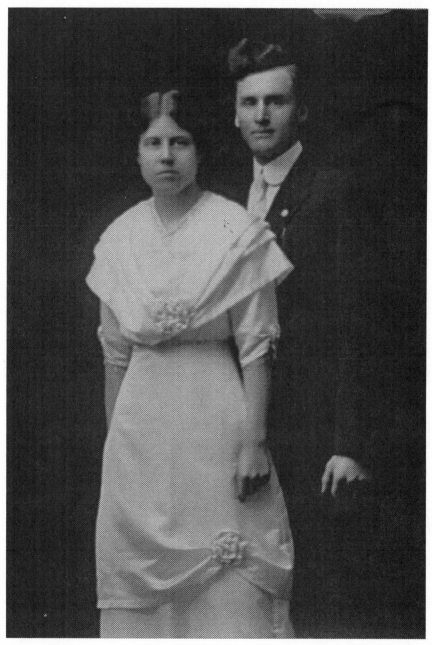

Virginian Alvin Miller Grove and his Indiana bride, Kathryn Everhock, who were married on December 13, 1913, in Millersburg, Indiana.

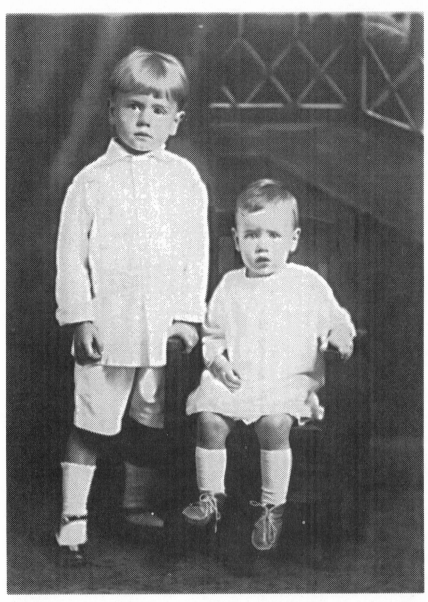

Ronald, age 3½, and Kedric, age 1½, two oldest children of Alvin and Kathryn Grove.

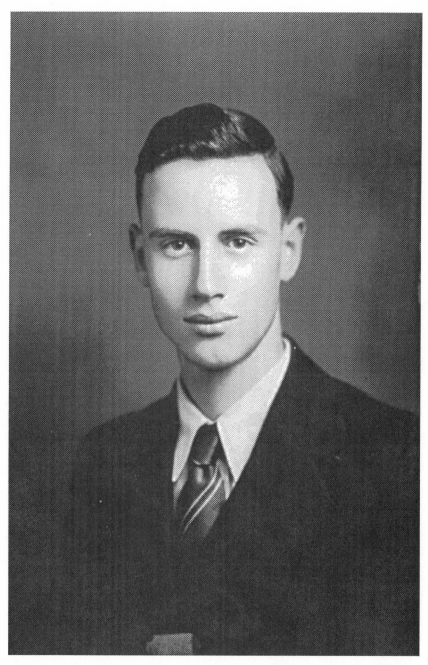

Kedric D. Grove, Bristol High School, Bristol, Indiana, Class of 1935.

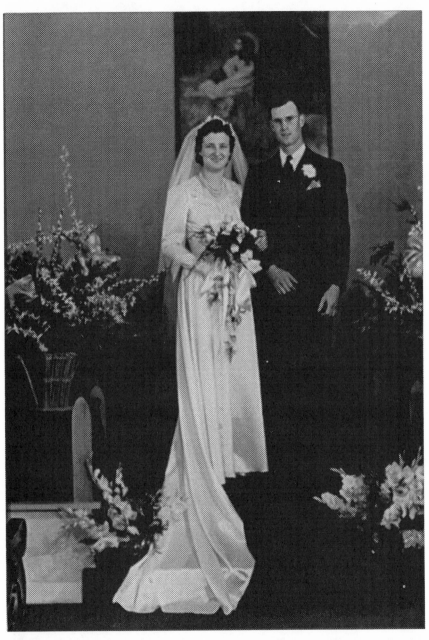

February 14, 1943, wedding of Kedric Grove and N. Florence Stombaugh in Bryan, Ohio.

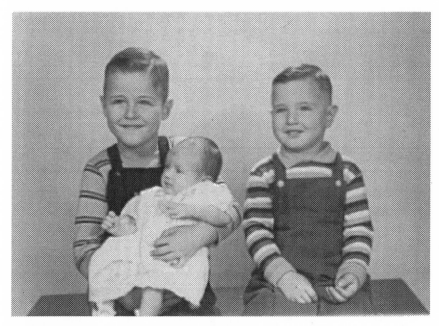

Children of Kedric and Florence Grove, taken in the early 1950s, with Dean, holding his sister Myrna, and Milan.

Chapter 4
Just Being My Dad

Dad's frame was thin and solid, and he weighed about 165 pounds. Because he often did manual work, his muscular arms could lift loads without strain. Despite his seventy years of age, he held his six foot height erect.

His hairline followed the Grove tradition of graying and receding. He grew sideburns to add to the band of hair around his head and the lack of it on top. He cleverly parted his hair on the side and combed strands across, giving the illusion of more hair.

Dad smiled in a kind way. His eyes twinkled as thoughts darted through his mind. Brown-framed glasses covered the upper part of his face. His dark, stubbly whiskers sometimes caused him to shave twice a day.

Dad was disinterested in fashionable dressing. While never dressed sloppily, he contented himself by wearing a pair of shoes for years. He constantly wore the same shirts. In the house or outside in the yard, he preferred denim work overalls and comfortable cotton shirts. He seldom shopped for new items, and sometimes we literally forced a new shirt or tie on him. It wasn't a matter of money, but a matter of keeping things until they wore out. Despite this trait, he dressed appropriately. However, Mom often checked to see that he wasn't wearing mismatched plaids.

My sociable father was mild-mannered, thoughtful, and curious. In his family, his mother raised him as her middle child. Perhaps his easygoing friendliness resulted from this placement. He seemed to take things as they came, seldom becoming upset or discouraged. Dad dealt with situations systematically as he reasoned things out. He liked to compare persons, not in a negative way, but just as observations. And he always greeted people he met and remembered details about them.

In a group situation, Dad would heartily introduce himself to nearly everyone present. He would converse with someone to find out whom they knew in common. Perhaps another person was related to his second cousin or had a brother who was unusually tall. He filed these curious facts away for use at future gatherings.

And questions erupted from him. He could ask several in a row, and then answer his own questions. Or, he answered one question with another. I puzzled about this method of communication, which was really a form of thinking aloud. Unless he directed a question to me, I seldom answered, but just listened.

I was unaware of my father's concept of illness since he had always been healthy. I knew that Dad had missed fewer than nine or ten days of work during his thirty year tenure at the General Motors Foundry. When he did have a cold, he never took medication. He preferred describing his symptoms rather than masking them with medicine.

In ice, rain, or snow, Dad departed on the eighteen mile, early morning drive from Bryan to the foundry in Defiance. The two towns were located in neighboring counties. He plodded to work during Ohio's blizzards of 1977 and 1978, following company policy that upon arrival, there would be work to do. He prided himself on his accountability.

During the 1978 blizzard, the foundry did close down. Already at work, Dad was unable to return home. He spent an uncomfortable night sleeping on three folding chairs and eating donuts and coffee. Finally, my parents' neighbor drove his four-wheeler over the snow-covered roads to rescue Dad.

Dad never made morning appearances as I was growing up. He would shower and go to bed about 10:00 P.M. His alarm woke him at four in the morning, and he shaved, cooked breakfast, and left long before the rest of the family awakened.

I do recall that when he came home late in the afternoon, his denim overalls were covered with light colored dust. Because of their condition, he removed his clothes and changed outfits as soon as he stepped inside the back door. He hung all his work clothes in a closet by the garage. Dust also covered his steel-toed shoes. He carried his special safety glasses in a case.

Dad had applied to work at General Motors after first farming for a living. For seven years, my parents rented farmland and animals on three different farms near Bryan, Ohio. They raised general crops such as corn, oats, wheat, alfalfa, and soybeans. Half of the profit from the crops, cattle, and chickens went to the farms' owners to pay for use of the land and the farmhouse. This arrangement did not prove very profitable for a young family. My parents couldn't get ahead financially.

Therefore, Dad applied for work at the General Motors Foundry in Defiance which had recently opened. Upon being hired in June of 1950, Dad began working third shift. From the beginning of Dad's association with General Motors, he was assigned to the core room. He was thirty-three years old. Immediately, fellow workers nicknamed him "Farmer."

Chapter 5
Looking for Hope

During the busy month of May, 1989, Dad barely found time to schedule his follow-up doctor's appointment. He was attending plays and concerts with my mother, and they were making summer plans. The middle of May arrived when he finally arranged for the CAT scan.

The May CAT scan showed that the soft tissue density on the right lung was slightly larger since the previous exam. Also, pleural thickening on the back of the right lung appeared more prominent. Again, the doctor recommended a biopsy of the right lung. Indeed, the mass had grown larger, not only in one, but in two locations.

Near the end of May, Dad returned as an outpatient for a biopsy of both questionable areas. He scheduled it between other events, including dental implants.

On a Tuesday evening, the surgeon called Dad at home. It was May 30, 1989, four months since his first suspicious checkup. The surgeon confirmed that the right lung biopsy, this time with a larger specimen, had tested positive for cancerous cells. The doctor advised Dad to come in for a consultation as soon as possible.

Sometimes denial is a useful tool. Such news is incomprehensible and difficult to fathom on a personal basis. Dad had never smoked, felt no physical symptoms, and led an active, clean lifestyle. Such a diagnosis seemed unreasonable. There was no family history of cancer on either side. Cancer just wasn't a diagnosis we expected to hear.

My parents cushioned themselves against the news. They busied themselves making arrangements for a Sunday School class party the next evening. Besides, the news had come at an inconvenient time. In less than two weeks, we were planning to fly to Seattle to attend my nephew Jason's high school graduation. And at the end of June, we hoped to fly to Orlando, Florida, for our church denomination's national conference. My parents had missed very few of these annual church meetings in the past thirty years.

For me, the last week of the school year, which is always an energy-taxing time, approached. I needed to complete year-end records and reports, besides coping daily with students who are anticipating summer vacation. Also, I had scheduled a weekend trip to Washington, D.C.

After school that Tuesday evening, I did some errands before driving to my parents' home. When I casually walked in the back door, they were preoccupied. Mom talked on the kitchen phone, as Dad watched television in the den. Dad came into the kitchen during a commercial and he smiled at me. I mentioned several things to him, including our upcoming trip to Seattle.

Dad patiently listened, and after I spoke, he calmly said, "The doctor called today, Myrna...he says it's a malignant cancer. I have to go in for another appointment. Something will have to be done about it soon."

I felt dumbfounded, as we looked at each other. Dad quickly turned away and went back to watch television while Mom continued on the phone. I slowly pulled out a chair to sit down. This pressing news took priority. Dad's health report isn't going to be so easy after all, I thought.

My cancer education was beginning. Roles in our family would never again be the same. One of the first things I learned was that cancer not only invades the life of the victim, but the lives of family members as well. Cancer becomes a way of life. There is the question of what to do next. And one is always looking for a ray of hope. The uncertainties about what is happening to a loved one can be very stressful.

I knew little about cancer, except that it seemed to be affecting more persons especially at younger ages. In recent years, several women friends had suffered breast cancer and had received successful treatments. I vaguely recalled their descriptions of the energy-sapping ordeal of chemotherapy and radiation.

What I knew about cancer of the lung was sparse. I had assumed that most victims were smokers. I was hoping that my father had just one little spot that could be removed surgically. After all, the spot had barely been visible four months before. I would assume an encouraging role with my parents and not promote undue worry.

Dad and Mom met with the local surgeon who explained that the cancer cells were consistent with poorly differentiated squamous cell carcinoma. (The doctor's assumption later turned out to be incorrect. Carcinoma is the most common cancer with solid tumors originating in a major organ rather than connective tissue, muscles, or bones.) The doctor recommended further CAT scans of the head, the bones, and the abdomen to find out how far the cancer had spread. He also spoke about surgery as an immediate possibility.

I had intended to be present at this appointment with the surgeon. Instead, as I headed toward the medical center, I met my parents' oncoming car. I had tried to leave school early and had been delayed. How could they be on their way home already? I wondered. Hadn't they asked any questions? Seeing me, they pulled over, and I joined them in their car.

Further CAT scans would take place Friday, and results would be back the following Monday, they explained matter-of-factly. It was a scary thought, indeed, to be looking in other locations for the cancer. Waiting for results could cause a worrisome weekend.

What would we do about our trip to Seattle? If Dad needed surgery right away, we wouldn't be able to go to Jason's graduation. How could we change our tickets at this late date? We were not thinking clearly.

We decided to ask the travel agent about possibilities under these new circumstances. The agent said that we would need to pay an additional sum on each ticket. Perhaps we could still leave on the original date and return home early for Dad's surgery. Maybe we shouldn't go at all. While we confused the travel agent with our dilemma, Mom couldn't remember where she had put the tickets. Thus, we accomplished nothing that evening.

During the next few months, this pattern of not knowing what to do or even whether it was possible continued. Plans could never be confirmed because we never knew in advance what my father's condition would be.

Meanwhile, my brother Dean, a physician near Seattle, Washington, made his own plans for our father. It was difficult for Dean to hear this unwelcome news and be so distant. Of course, Dean still wanted us to come for his son's graduation. Because he did not have a clear picture of what was happening, Dean suggested to Mom and Dad that they come to the Swedish Medical Center Hospital and its leading cancer center in Seattle for a second opinion.

As a doctor, my brother made referrals to Swedish Hospital and had connections to staff members. Dean could arrange for preliminary tests, further biopsies, and consultations. The Tumor Institute, as it is called, dealt frequently with many kinds of cancer diagnoses. Its doctors did thoracotomies, or surgeries of the chest, frequently. My father was soon convinced that the Seattle doctors could check him, and possibly perform the necessary surgery.

My sister-in-law Mary worked out the logistics of the Seattle flights. She discovered that for medical emergencies, the airline could leave our return flight open-ended. My father could then stay in Seattle for surgery or opt to return to Ohio.

During the weekend after my father's CAT scans, I had been in Washington, D.C. While I was gone, the impending results weighed heavily on my mind. On Monday, Bryan's hospital reported that Dad's head, bone, and abdomen scans appeared to be clear of cancer. We welcomed the news.

The local medical center agreed to send copies of reports, X-rays, and slides with us to give the doctors in Seattle. I felt relief that there would now be a second opinion and that my brother would assist in planning what to do. His medical knowledge and personal care would be a great asset in dealing with Dad's problems. We packed our bags quickly for the trip to the Northwest.

Chapter 6
A Weekend Reprieve

The evening we arrived in Seattle, my brother delivered Dad's X-rays to his neighbor who was on staff at Swedish Hospital as a radiologist. Late the same night, the radiologist read the X-rays. Then, Dean scheduled three days of consultations and tests for Dad, beginning Monday morning. Normally, this much testing would require about two weeks to carry out. But time was important, and Dean was able to make the plans efficiently.

In the meantime, we could rest and enjoy the weekend. A special graduation dinner was on the agenda for Jason, Dean's younger son. Our family savored my sister-in-law's culinary expertise, and both sets of Jason's grandparents watched with pride as he opened gifts. Jason was enrolled at the University of Washington as a freshman. He received typical graduation items including a typewriter, luggage, a study lamp, and money.

Derek, Dean's older son, was home from his second year at Washington State University. With him, he had brought an unexpected summer guest, his fraternity's mascot dog. Maddie, a black Newfoundland, bore the size and shape of a black grizzly bear. She ambled around the house giving friendly gazes and getting chased from off-limit rooms. It was amazing that she moved around without disturbing the household furnishings.

East Side Catholic High School held their Sunday evening commencement in the gymnasium of Bellevue Community College. We arrived in time to claim aisle seats on the main floor. About 200 seniors marched to the traditional "Pomp and Circumstance." Camera bulbs flashed to capture moments of entrance and the congratulatory handshakes.

After various awards, one of the speakers gave a brief speech using the text of Robert Fulghum's book, *All I Really Need to Know, I Learned in Kindergarten.* The speaker emphasized that what we learn to get us through life starts when we are very young, and some of the same basic principles still apply. As life gets more complicated, it's still important to work and play well with others, to delight in living, and to realize there is a cycle for all God's creatures.

To me, it seemed my nephew Jason, whose height at age seventeen towered at 6'4", had recently completed Peter Rabbit Nursery School. How had time passed so rapidly from that event to this one? What had happened to the passage of time between significant milestones in my family's life?

The summer weather was pleasant that weekend, and one could lay aside cares. My brother's family lived in a newly developed subdivision on a hill overlooking the Seattle skyline and Lake Washington. From their wooden deck, one could see bridges over waterways and a range of snow-covered Olympic Mountains. The houses were built on the hillside so they wouldn't obstruct neighbors' views. Wide glass windows opened toward the majestic scenery. Pine trees and deer nestled between houses along the winding road which led to the hill's summit.

Since Dad was still on his exercise regime, he and I walked around the neighborhood. The fresh pine smell and mountain landscapes enticed us. We would climb up the hillside and wind around nearby cul-de-sacs. Since blocks had no square corners, we would disagree on the route. The day before Dad's tests began, we got lost and probably walked an extra mile before asking directions. When we reached the house, we were both short of breath.

On Sunday evening, Mary brought out a marzipan-iced birthday cake to surprise Dad for a belated birthday party. In the confusion, we had missed Dad's 72nd birthday the previous week. We talked and laughed and ate cake at the kitchen table. In my card, I wished Dad happiness on this birthday and on all the ones to come. The possibility that this might be his last birthday crossed my mind.

We were up early Monday morning. Dean wanted to leave before the morning rush hour traffic across the Mercer Island Bridge to Seattle. Since the procedures to be done were in several different buildings, I was to accompany Dad rather than tax my mother's walking. Dean would stay with us or be one step ahead, when necessary. I was prepared, notebook in hand, for the first appointment.

Chapter 7
Seeking a Diagnosis

The next three days were a whirlwind of medical appointments with Dad as an outpatient. Some occurred in the early morning, and some took place late at night. We found that a city hospital is open at all hours.

Swedish Hospital itself was a complex of stone buildings near downtown Seattle. Walkways and elevators connected the tall structures and the parking garage. It challenged us to find the right medical department on the appropriate floor.

Even though the exterior was massive in size, the interior invited personal friendliness. The pleasing, modern decor was soothing. Airy, green plants and urns of hot water for coffee and tea were placed in the waiting areas, and there were small coffee shops on walkways between buildings. A large cafeteria, popular with staff as well as visitors, sported a cappuccino bar in one corner. Everything about the hospital promoted comfort, and for two weeks, it would be our second home.

First, we went to a waiting room on the main floor to enroll Dad in the hospital's computer. Dad related details of his life history and provided proof of medical coverage to the receptionist, as he remembered facts with ease. Once registered, he was ready to begin his tests.

Mostly, I was able to stay with Dad. I felt this was important since he was experiencing his first hospital visit in a new environment with an uncertain outcome. I began to note our role reversals, me becoming the guiding parent and my father becoming the trusting child. We followed my brother's chronological list of appointments.

Dad's first appointment was for a biopsy of the lower back lobe on his right lung. It was done using CAT scan guidance. While partially covered by a sheet, Dad lay on his stomach with the imposing computer X-ray machine stationed above him. He rolled in various positions while doctors studied a cross-sectional view of his chest. My brother and I watched the screen in an adjoining room.

The doctor pointed out the thickened chest wall, visible on the CAT scan. It was difficult for me to distinguish, but the doctors all agreed. Next, the doctor used a needle to biopsy the lower right lobe. Displeased with the first specimen, the doctor did two more biopsies. Then, he sent the tissue to the lab for analysis.

Next, the hospital lab, open twenty-four hours a day, took blood samples. Giving blood would become second nature to Dad as his ordeal continued.

Late the same day, our family met with an oncologist at the Tumor Institute. He was a low-key, congenial man. At nine o'clock in the evening, patients waited to consult with him. He must be very dedicated, I thought, and he realizes the urgency in a cancer patient's time schedule.

The doctor himself greeted us and escorted us to the consultation room. About fifty years in age, he was thin in stature with slightly receding, sandy-colored hair. We immediately trusted his unassuming manner. On the receptionist's desk, I noticed a doll figurine which appeared to be a medical doctor in motion with coat tails, stethoscope, and hair flying behind it. Its inscription thanked the doctor for his care during cancer treatments. I assumed it was a gift from a patient.

In the consultation, Dad told the results of his physical exam five months before. Then, he recited the scenario of the May cancer diagnosis.

The oncologist asked Dad about his medical history. The only surgery my father could recall was a tonsillectomy at age five which the family doctor had performed on the kitchen table during a house call. Dad revealed that he was a non-smoker and had lost about ten pounds in recent months. He attributed the weight loss to exercise and diet. Most of his answers were negative regarding possible ailments.

I listened intently as Dad told his family's medical history. His father had died twenty-five years before of myocardial infarction and hypertension. His mother had died a year later of renal kidney failure. Dad's older brother had died of a heart attack. Because of this history, Dad watched his diet and faithfully kept track of his cholesterol level. Dad was proud of these preventative health measures.

My parents' history included two sons and a daughter, in their late thirties and early forties, who had no unusual physical problems. Mother, at age seventy-three, had only a slight limp from childhood polio and some allergies for which she took shots. Dad's sixty-four year old sister had previously doctored for angina.

In response to possible injuries or exposures, Dad told how he was exposed to dust and smoke on a daily basis during his employment at the foundry. The doctor noted this on the chart, as well as the presence of a mild cough and slight hearing decrease.

Upon examination, the oncologist found Dad's blood pressure and heart sinus rhythm to be normal. The doctor's impression was that Dad had a localized, non-small cell cancer of the right lung. He would need further tests before surgery was set.

More tests were scheduled the second day. These included a pleural fluid thoracentesis with ultrasound and a pulmonary function test to determine blood gas levels. While going to and from tests, we had little time to think about their purpose and impact.

The thoracentesis was an examination of the chest by ultrasound and a withdrawal of pleural fluid by needle. The doctors examined both the right and left chest. During ultrasound, tumor tissue causes a different echo than normal tissue. No problems were detected on Dad's left side.

However, a small pleural effusion of 1-2 cm excess fluid was apparent on the right side. The pleural thickening was again visible. The doctor removed 90 cc's of fluid for the lab to study, and then sent Dad for a chest X-ray.

The chest X-ray showed a nodular pleural thickening along the right lateral surface. This meant little to me as one rarely thinks about having problems in the pleura. I thought his problem was in the lung. Whoever heard of having cancer in the chest lining? Hopefully, the areas were confined to the right side, I thought.

Dad performed in the pulmonary function test by blowing into a machine called a spirometer. The doctor said his flow rates were moderately reduced by a slight constriction in his bronchial tubes with no significant trapped air. Blood gases in the arteries and atmospheric pressure in his blood both tested normal.

The lab reported that Monday's biopsy of the lower right pleura was benign. The examining doctor was not sure if the tumor was in the lung or if it could be a "mesothelioma" in the lining of the lung. The doctor's conjecture of mesothelioma held no reference for me.

Tuesday's agenda also involved meeting with the thoracic surgeon. The interview is an opportunity for the surgeon to assess the patient's general health and his fitness for surgery. He also answers any pertinent questions the patient may have. My family met with the surgeon in a medical building adjacent to the hospital.

The surgeon was a confident, pleasant-mannered man. He was about fifty-five with medium-brown, well-coifed hair. He spoke forthrightly about the upcoming surgery as a needed tool for a definitive diagnosis. He professionally described surgery as a logical, everyday occurrence which he could competently handle.

The surgeon explained how a thoracotomy, or opening of the chest in hopes of finding the problem, would require about three-and-a-half hours. During this time, a ventilator would do Dad's breathing for him instead of his lungs. During surgery, the doctor would freeze the nerves from the spine to the chest wall. This freezing would cut back on post-surgical pain. After being numbed, the nerves usually don't grow back for about a year. After being in the recovery room for about two hours, Dad would have a hospital stay of a week and a recuperation at home for another week.

During the interview, the surgeon asked Dad about his work exposures. The doctor noted that Dad had worked in a foundry for many years. He also discovered that Dad had been a non-smoker. The doctor wondered if Dad could possibly have been exposed to some amount of asbestos at the foundry. Dad responded that he had never given much thought to it.

By this time, we were all anxious about Dad's problem. The sooner it could be taken care of, the better. The doctor was reassuring, and before we left the office, Dad agreed to surgery. The surgeon scheduled it for the coming Thursday, two days hence.

Later in the afternoon, Dad went to the Tumor Institute to discuss his participation in Protocol 8810, a non-small cell antibody scan. The scan itself was not a treatment, but it was an experimental means of detecting cancer cells in the body which might not be visible by normal X-ray and CAT scan.

An oncology nurse was in charge of explaining the study and getting Dad's consent as a participant. She said the test had been used in research for three years. The X-ray is safe and has about the same radiation exposure as a regular bone scan.

If Dad agreed to the protocol, a radio-labeled infusion, or a fluid marker designed to concentrate in certain cells to potentially identify other sites of tumor, would be injected later the same evening. The nurse would note vital signs and monitor Dad for an hour before sending him home.

The actual X-ray would be done the following morning, using

circular cameras at various angles. The radioactive substance would enhance the X-ray and cause cancer cells in the body to light up. The X-ray process would require about two hours. The infusion would leave the body in 14-17 hours. For a 24-hour period after infusion, Dad would have to save his urine. And for the next few months, he would need to send blood samples to the Tumor Institute to see if antibodies were stimulated or if he had had a harmful reaction. Dad agreed to be in the research protocol.

After a day of tests, Dad returned in the evening for the antibody scan infusion. He tolerated it without incident, and he was excited to be part of a research project.

On Wednesday morning, Dad received the actual X-ray for the antibody scan. He was given a schedule for follow-up blood samples along with tubes to mail them which the local medical center in Ohio would need. In six months, when Dad returned to Seattle, a re-scanning could be done.

The final day of tests included an EKG and CAT scans of the chest, abdomen, and pelvis. The chest scan showed the same pleural based lesion on the right lower back. No lesions were found in the liver or spleen. The adrenals, kidneys, and pancreas were normal. According to the scans, the cancer had not spread to other organs.

On the day before surgery, the doctor received a pathology report on the pleural fluid. The evaluation revealed small bland cells which were twice the diameter of a lymphocyte. The cells were of uncertain origin and appeared to be benign.

My father had tolerated the tests with a determined spirit, and we had supported him throughout with our presence and words of encouragement. From the battery of tests prior to surgery, the doctors could not make a conclusive diagnosis.

Chapter 8
Anticipating Tomorrow

After the third day of tests, we went home to my brother's house, exhausted. It seemed that every potential organ in my father had been probed and scanned. I knew my way around the medical center like an employee.

Summer was usually a time of recuperation from the school year. But before having a break, my family was facing serious decisions about Dad on the opposite side of the country. I was present out of love and concern for my father, and I wanted him to receive the best care available.

Events leading to surgery had happened rapidly, as if life was suddenly on fast forward. Dad had always been healthy and strong. He had put his family first and been faithful in his love and support, even after his three offspring had grown to adulthood. And Dad and Mom had traveled to each coast two or three times a year to visit their four grandsons. Two grandsons lived near Seattle, and two lived near Philadelphia. Keeping up with their grandchildren's activities had been important to them.

Mom depended on Dad for many things. His hand held her steady when they walked. He attended to paying the bills. Dad did physical jobs around the house such as lifting, carrying, and moving. He made lists about errands.

I hadn't considered my parents' vulnerability. I thought they would always be here. Even though independent from them, it comforted me to know they were nearby enjoying life.

I hoped the surgery would be a positive step toward a continuing, active lifestyle. I knew how hard my parents had worked. That's why I was glad their recent years of retirement had been carefree and healthy. They had just completed payment of their thirty-year home mortgage. The ranch-style house had been built to their specifications, and in 1959, they had moved into the new country home with their young family. More recently, Dad had constructed a two-story hip roof barn behind the house. Built with his own hands, the barn was an art form and a source of great pride.

There were more places that Mom and Dad wanted to travel. They had already visited every state including Alaska and Hawaii. They had toured Europe several times with special groups. Their most memorable trip had been to the Holy Land, Greece, and Egypt. Dad spoke about wanting to visit Australia next.

During the medical tests, Dean had told Dad that he didn't necessarily have to go through surgery or follow-up treatments. He could stop at any time if he chose. Of course, a diagnosis would be difficult without the surgery. However, Dean wanted Dad to know that he had options, and doctors could not dictate to him. Dean also wanted Dad to know that all the medical procedures might not make a difference in the final outcome.

Dad always elected to continue treating the cancer. This surprised me somewhat because of Dad's lack of medical experience. But he still believed cancer was a disease to fight, an illness he wished to rally against. Sickness had never been a part of his daily life.

I barely slept the night before Dad's surgery. After my family returned from the anointing service, we talked about trivial issues, striving to be positive. I reminded Dad that the anesthesia would cause him to sleep through half a day or more. We were hopeful before hugging him good night. We were taking each day as it came.

Chapter 9
Waiting for Answers

The morning of surgery arrived. At sunrise, we greeted the day and boarded our van for the hospital in time for a 6:00 A.M. admission. We were the first ones in the surgical patients' ward, and Dad was assigned to the only private room available. After Dad undressed and put on a hospital gown, we gathered around his bed.

Minutes dragged by. The red-headed nurse on duty greeted us cheerfully as she took care of preliminaries. Her name tag read "Toy." She asked the official list of questions for patients. Hearing Dad's answers, one would think he was perfectly well because to each question he obediently responded, "No."

When the nurse finished with the list of ailments, she laughingly countered, "Well, if nothing is wrong with you, what are you doing here?"

To this, Dad replied, "You haven't asked me if I have cancer." Indeed, she hadn't.

While making rounds, the surgeon came in briefly. He was calm and supportive. After telling us the schedule for surgery, he added that Dad would soon be given a shot to make him drowsy. Dad wondered who would be assisting during surgery, and the doctor mentioned the anesthesiologist and others. Then, still wearing his street clothes, the doctor departed on further rounds.

Shortly before the 9:00 A.M. surgery, orderlies arrived to wheel Dad to the surgery room on the lower level. They hoisted him from the bed to the gurney, and we followed them to the hall. Since only one person could go with him, we decided it should be Mom.

I hadn't been able to speak at the anointing service the evening before, and I hadn't said much that morning. If I remained silent, my chances might be gone. "I love you, Dad," I whispered, as the gurney rolled down the hall.

"I know you do, Myrna," Dad replied as he reached up to touch my arm. Then, he was wheeled away. I was relieved that Dad had known all along how much I loved him, even when it was unspoken.

Another orderly escorted us to the main lobby which also served as the surgical waiting area. There was enough activity there to keep families occupied and distracted. My sister-in-law and I claimed two cushioned chairs near a coffee urn and settled in. We had brought books to read. Mom returned to us shortly, and my brother would come back to the hospital later.

While waiting, I intended to read Bernie Siegel's bestseller, *Peace, Love, and Healing.* I wanted to find out what this cancer business was all about. I knew that Dr. Siegel wrote uplifting advice about dealing with cancer and what part the mind plays in healing the body. If a surgeon can acknowledge that a person's attitude aids his healing process, there must be some validity to it, I thought.

As the morning passed, I read several chapters as I contemplated how we might use Dr. Siegel's philosophy in our own situation. Once in a while, I looked up to watch people, and I noticed numerous children with bald heads or head coverings. The children are here for their cancer treatments, I concluded. How sad that they are struggling for life at such young ages.

The surgery seemed to be taking a long time. After stopping by his office that morning, my brother arrived to wait with us. Because we didn't want to miss the doctor when he came out of surgery, we remained in the lobby past lunchtime.

It was nearly 1:30 P.M. when the doctor emerged wearing his green surgical gown. Seeing us, he came over to sit on the stool in front of us. His face looked serious.

"I don't have very good news," he said. He paused and then continued, "When we opened the chest area, we found not only the thickened pleura, but multiple tumor involvement on the diaphragm." My mind was swimming. The surgeon went on as if we were comprehending his words. "The lesion on the upper lobe extended both into the lung and into the chest wall. Such thickened pleura is rather typical for mesothelioma, a cancerous condition brought on by exposure to asbestos."

"We don't know that he has been exposed to asbestos," Mom retorted.

"Well, somewhere along the line, he has been," the surgeon replied, while we looked at him numbly.

He continued with his findings. "During surgery, the pleura was stripped from the chest wall. Samples were taken from the diaphragm, but since there was extensive tumor elsewhere in the pleura, we did not remove the diaphragm." I hoped my brother understood all of this.

"We did remove the bulky tumor on the upper chest and clipped the area to outline it for radiotherapy," the surgeon added. "However, it was impossible to find and remove all the tumors because of the way this cancer seeds itself around the chest." He paused.

"I wish I had better news to tell you," the doctor apologized. My mother was leaning forward from her chair on her knees. My brother's face looked pale white. This is impossible, I thought. It was just one little spot, wasn't it, maybe two? Dad hadn't even had any symptoms.

I foolishly blurted out questions which didn't really have answers. "How long does he have?" I asked.

"Typically, other persons with this disease have lived twelve to eighteen months," he replied. Any limitation now seemed to me like too short a time. The doctor was hesitant to give exact times, but rather meant that there was no cure and the disease was progressive.

"Will it be very painful when the tumors grow?" I asked, wanting to protect my father from this sudden curse.

"With medication and treatment, the pain level can be reduced. I froze the nerves above and below the incision, and this should be of some help. He lost very little blood and did not need a transfusion. He'll be coming out of the recovery room before too long," the doctor concluded. Then, he excused himself while we were left to cope with our reactions.

I could hardly pronounce the name of the diagnosis. Meso... meso...meso...what? I hadn't wanted the answers to my impulsive questions. What would we do now? Dad had been so hopeful about coming to this cancer center. And now, we received this news. What does asbestos have to do with it? It was too unbelievable to assimilate, like a bad dream.

My sister-in-law looked at my tear-stained face and gave me a hug. "Let it out," she said. I was uncomfortable reacting to the news in public. I hadn't wanted to cry, but the news was just so unexpected.

My brother suggested that we get some lunch in the cafeteria while Dad was in the recovery room, but eating hardly appealed to me. Dean tried to be cheerful with Mom. "We'll have to hear what the oncologist says about treatment and go from there," he advised. Silently, we rode the elevator to the basement.

In the cafeteria, I selected a health food sandwich. My brother smiled weakly at me as we sat down to eat. "Are you okay?" he asked.

Instead of answering, I got up and ran out of the room. I didn't want to be around other people. I found the ladies' restroom down the hall, went in, and burst into tears. This irrational behavior was untypical for me. I tried to wash my face so it would be less puffy when I emerged from my self-imposed cocoon. Our lives had taken an unexpected turn.

Chapter 10
Rallying Toward Recovery

Later in the afternoon, we went to see Dad in intensive care. We prepared ourselves for the worst, expecting his body to be a freeway of tubes and bandages. As we entered his room, however, Dad looked surprisingly perky. He was sitting up in bed, eating a full-course chicken dinner and watching television. He smiled warmly at us.

I wondered why there was such a contrast between the prognosis and Dad's cheerful mood. Perhaps there had been a mistake. After all, the lab hadn't analyzed the surgery biopsies yet. I found out later that the surgeon had said he would talk to Dad about the surgery when Dad was more alert. I'm sure Dad was just glad the surgery was over. I wondered if he should be eating so much after the anesthesia.

A male nurse arrived just in time to rescue the dessert from Dad's ravenous appetite. He hadn't expected Dad to feel like eating and had forgotten to suggest a limited intake. Poor Dad had missed regular meals during the past four days.

Dad stayed in intensive care overnight before moving to a private room on the seventh floor which had a view of Mount Rainier. They think of everything at this hospital, I thought, admiring the outdoor scene. We spent the hospital days sitting beside Dad while he rested. Often, we would sit and read rather than talk. Mother did crossword puzzles. Each of us had his own way of coping.

By the second day after surgery, the doctor suggested Dad get up and walk. "It's a cruel world," the doctor laughingly advised.

Of course, this meant that Dad had to take his IVs and catheter with him. We pushed the pole-like contraptions as we walked a circular path around the halls. I held Dad's free hand. It was quite a contrast to the walks we had taken near my brother's house just the week before.

One day, Mary brought Dad a bowl of fresh strawberries which he heartily ate. The comparison between the hospital menu and fresh strawberries had been tempting. But she had not intended for him to eat them all at once. Later, Dad regretted the urgent problem their ingestion had caused. He forgot to request assistance as he hurried to the bathroom. In his weakened condition, he fell down and bumped his head. The experience reminded him to ask for help when he needed it. After all, his independent lifestyle was being curtailed.

Chest drain tubes protruded from the surgical wounds. The oncologist decided to give Dad some cisplatinum chemotherapy directly through these tubes. One evening, we left early so the procedure could be done.

The cisplatinum was administered while Dad was rocked to and fro, even sideways and upside down on the bed. This movement made certain the chemo completely coated the chest cavity and came in contact with as many cancer cells as possible. In the process, Dad was given medicine to protect his kidneys and to prevent nausea.

The combinations and amounts of medication caused Dad to hallucinate. He later described evil creatures who were having meetings around him and driving big cars. He knew it was the medication, and yet he could watch them from the corner of his eye. It was an unpleasant sight until the medication wore off. The next day I told him that if it happened again, we would call Ghostbusters!

Dad received special attention from hospital staff. The chief of staff encouraged us by saying that the initial treatment is sometimes the most important. My brother's colleague brought a care package. And the minister who had done the anointing service stopped periodically for a visit and prayer.

Dad received daily phone calls from my brother in Philadelphia and from friends and relatives in Ohio. We arranged his cards on the shelf above his television.

It seemed odd to see a circle of staples down Dad's back and side. Apparently, the 15-inch incision enclosed with metal staples was not as uncomfortable as it looked, and it was just as conducive to healing. Dad was a cooperative and energetic patient. The recovery week passed swiftly, and he was released on the sixth day after surgery. Before he left, the staples were removed.

Dad returned to Dean's home for another restful week of recovery. Further appointments were scheduled with the oncologist and the surgeon. Dad and I resumed our daily walks, but this time we didn't climb the steeper hills, and I held Dad's hand to support him.

Shortly after that, Mary invited a neighbor for brunch. The woman, in her forties, was a friend and a professional counselor whom Mary had recently assisted. Mary now thought that Dad could share his feelings with someone. This particular woman could not only listen to Dad, but closely associate with his fears. In the past few months, she herself had undergone a double mastectomy with extensive cancer involvement in the lymph nodes. Her cancer had appeared without much warning. She experienced complications after surgery and was in the midst of chemotherapy treatments while still working with patients and taking care of her family. She talked patiently with Dad and told him about her initial denial of the diagnosis and how she was forced to deal with it. Because I had my own trouble coping, I wasn't anxious to hear about someone else. In his sociable way, Dad seemed to converse with her very well. I admired this woman for her courage, and I thought it ironic that, in her state, she was the one comforting us.

Chapter 11
Consulting with the Oncologist

Two days after his hospital release, Dad met with the oncologist at the Tumor Institute. Once the oncologist was available, he gave us his undivided attention. Dad pointed out a fluid build-up near his incision. The doctor said that as the scar contracts, the tissue hangs over, but the excess would eventually go away.

"How effective was the cisplatinum treatment?" Mom wondered.

"We don't know," the doctor replied, "but anything we can do to help mesothelioma, we'll try. We used a high concentration of cisplatinum in a small area."

Dad asked, "Does this kind of cancer spread out of the chest cavity very fast?"

"There are two kinds of mesothelioma," stated the doctor, "one that grows fast and one that grows slowly. We don't know which kind you have until later. You've probably had this for six months. There's no way of knowing."

The doctor continued, "You're a non-smoker with mesothelioma. You could be compensated."

"What you're saying is if I picked it up due to environmental conditions where I worked, there's a way you get compensated for your injury?" Dad questioned.

"Yes, you and your family," the doctor answered.

"We haven't thought about pursuing that," said my brother.

Mom struggled with her notes, "Can you spell the kind of cancer he has?"

"It's mesothelioma," the doctor repeated. "I'll write it down."

Then, the doctor asked Dad, "How's your stamina?"

"Pretty good," Dad answered. "I could make somebody flinch if I wanted to. I've been walking two or three blocks twice a day. I don't have any problems with my legs or getting out of breath."

"You can walk as much as you want to," the doctor advised.

"Are there any cancer doctors in Bryan?"

"There's an oncologist affiliated with the medical center," Dean answered.

The doctor then inquired about cities close to Bryan which have oncology centers. We said that cancer patients usually go to Fort Wayne, Indiana, or Toledo, Ohio, for treatment. The doctor buzzed his nurse and asked her to find out what hospitals have membership in the Southwest Oncology Group (SWOG) network.

A nurse then delivered two protocol treatments for mesothelioma to the doctor. The first one was developed in 1981 and the second in 1984. A protocol, I soon learned, is a formal statement of a treatment regimen. The mesothelioma protocols included radiation with or without chemotherapy. Dad was already too old to participate in one of them which had very strict age guidelines.

Turning directly to Dad, the doctor said, "This disease is mainly in the pleura. With X-ray therapy, they can treat that area very nicely."

"Will the pleura repair itself — what they scraped away, will it repair itself in time?" Dad wanted to know.

"No," the doctor answered succinctly.

"You can also use interferon for treatment," he continued, "but you will get better care if your doctor back home chooses his own treatment. Here, we give ten milligrams of platinum a day, along with radiation, to sensitize the cells. Or, you can be on a national protocol. There's no wrong way of doing it, as long as you do well," concluded the doctor.

"Would radiation be started three or four weeks post-surgery?" my brother asked. The doctor replied affirmatively.

While flipping through the protocol pages, the doctor said, "It tells here that there's no cure for this disease."

Dad responded, "In other words, you would never test negative for these cells?"

The doctor turned to Dean, "Did anyone tell your Dad about this?" Dean said he thought the surgeon had.

"I thought radiation, in time, would knock these cells down and kill them off," Dad stated.

"Kill them off? I don't know if it can kill them all," replied the doctor.

"In other words, it's just like diabetes. You have to live with it, doctor it, and keep it under control?" Dad asked, hopefully.

Mary interjected, "The purpose is to slow it down. It's progressive."

"And how good a job we can do, we don't know," added the doctor.

"Some kinds of cancer can be arrested, but this isn't that way?" asked Dad.

"This is a more malignant type of cancer," the doctor agreed.

Mom asked, "Is it because of lack of research in this area?"

The doctor explained, "We usually can only detect the disease when the tumors are too far advanced. That's the major problem. There's only one lady I know of who was cured. Her abdominal mesothelioma was discovered accidentally during surgery for something else, before it had spread. That was ten to fifteen years ago."

Mary asked, "Does attitude have anything to do with it?"

"Yes," the doctor responded, "and your Dad has a super attitude."

Dad asked, "Will radiation keep it from spreading?"

"Radiation should really knock it out and stunt it for a long period of time. But once you've had radiation in a certain area, you're done. Then, you have to use other things to fight it, such as different kinds of chemotherapy," explained the doctor.

"Will radiation slow down your everyday life?" Dad asked.

"Yes, it will poop you out. You will have to rest. It's like being out in the sun too long. The first week or so, you'll be a little tired, and week by week, you'll get progressively more tired," the doctor clarified.

"After you quit for a while and your strength comes back, can you go out and work right along with everybody?" Dad asked.

"In two or three months," the doctor responded.

We were waiting for the nurse to return with contacts in Ohio who were members of SWOG. We discussed possible locations for treatment and the advantages and disadvantages. Suggestions included Ann Arbor, Detroit, Indianapolis, Fort Wayne, Columbus, and Toledo, which all had oncology treatment centers.

"Is here in Washington an option?" Mary wondered.

"Toledo would be my first choice," Dad stated, "if anyone there is capable. It's much closer than having to live somewhere else. I'd be more satisfied, you know."

"What kind of schedule are we looking at?" asked Dean.

"It's six weeks daily," the doctor answered.

Then, the doctor inserted his own personal message about his mother's ovarian cancer fifteen years before. He said she spent three months in Houston getting the best radiotherapy available, and today, she's fine.

Choosing the right place is difficult, I thought, and might even determine the outcome. Considering Dad's comfort and needs, where would the best place be? I wondered.

While we waited, the doctor called Columbus to inquire about recommended cancer centers. He explained that he had a patient from Ohio with malignant pleural mesothelioma who would be returning to Ohio for follow-up radiation treatments. He asked which locations had research centers and staff oncologists on hand, if a problem arose. I wondered how we would arrange accommodations if the treatment center was at a distance. The newest and most appropriate equipment seemed to be a necessary factor.

"Can they do that kind of pleural radiation in Toledo at Flower Hospital?" we overheard the doctor ask. "Is the equipment as good as Ohio State's?"

Now, I began to hope that Dad would get to sleep in his own bed at night during the six-week radiation treatment. Flower Hospital was located northwest of Toledo in the suburb of Sylvania, an hour's drive from Bryan.

Recently, I had visited a friend in physical therapy at the Lake Park Hospital and Nursing Care Center next to Flower Hospital. The hospital itself was an imposing stone structure which appeared to be fairly new. The buildings, set back from the road, were located behind two large duck ponds on either side of a curved drive.

"So you think Flower Hospital is as good as anywhere else?" we heard the doctor say. "Flower has the right equipment?"

After the doctor hung up, we soon decided on Flower Hospital. Dad was pleased with the decision.

"Do you have any words of wisdom on how to answer questions from others such as 'Did they get all the tumor?'" Mary asked intently. This concerned my mother.

"The truth...tell the truth," the doctor responded. "That's why you're having further treatments. The tumor's not all removed."

Regarding his diet, Dad wondered if he should watch his intake of fats. The doctor said that persons with cancer have decreased heart disease, probably because they eat less. "Eat everything you want," he suggested. "You will lose weight with the radiation."

The doctor directed us to see the oncologist in Sylvania as soon as we returned to Ohio. He said it takes at least a week to make preparations for the radiation. As we went out the door, the doctor added, "You've got a wonderful family."

"Thanks," Dad said, "you've been a real friend. See you at Christmastime."

Chapter 12
Follow-up with the Surgeon

A week later, Dad, Mom, and I met with the surgeon. Even though Dad complained of a deep tiredness in his chest, the surgeon thought he was doing well. The incision was healing, and Dad was sleeping well at night. Having avoided vigorous exercise, the doctor now told Dad to literally climb the walls with his fingers.

The surgeon asked about the plan for radiation. Dad told him that the oncologist had made contacts in Sylvania, and it was being set up there. The surgeon thought that sounded like a good solution.

"Would the radiation hit me on the front and the back, too?" Dad wondered.

"Well, there are two areas of concern," the surgeon said. "One is in front where the tumor was. We marked that with clips as a target area. The other place would be along the diaphragm. The diaphragm can be easily seen on film."

"There wouldn't have been an easy way to pinpoint the trouble without the operation, would there?" asked Dad.

The doctor answered, "Well, we had just tiny bits of tissue, and they have trouble making a diagnosis with that."

"And it would have been hard to get rid of the tumor in front with only radiation, wouldn't it?" Dad wanted to confirm.

The doctor responded, "Yes, the less tumor you have, the more effective radiation is. We didn't remove the chest wall or the nodules on the diaphragm. If there was one area, and we could take that out and say we're rid of the thing, then it's worth removing the diaphragm and putting in a replacement. But since there's no way to cure the problem with surgery, there's no point in putting you through the added risk. We can get it down in terms of size. We can find out exactly what it is, but we can't get rid of every cell."

Dad looked thoughtful, "Now, these cells aren't common like

51

lung cancer from cigarettes? It's very uncommon?"

The doctor replied, "It's a less common tumor by a long shot. It's caused by asbestos."

"The more I think about it," said Dad, "we had some asbestos boards at the plant which had another mineral with it. They were solid boards to lay on ovens, and we put cores on top of them. That was in the early days."

"Was that in the fifties?" I wondered. "When did they stop using it?"

"Well, they still had asbestos in some things. The ovens used to be insulated with asbestos." Then, Dad added, "The schools are spending a lot of money to take it out now. They didn't know about it 30-40 years ago. Furnace pipes used to be wrapped with asbestos to insulate them. Everybody's been exposed to a little."

"I think you told me you worked around pipes," the doctor stated.

"Well, it was just part of the ongoing work at the foundry where I would have gotten it," replied Dad.

"It doesn't seem to take a lot of exposure," the doctor interjected. "That's the thing about asbestos. And there's about a thirty year latent period before the tumor arises."

"Oh, I see," Dad said as if hearing this for the first time.

"Over in Bremerton across Puget Sound, we saw quite a bit of mesothelioma among shipyard workers thirty years after World War II," the doctor said.

"Was asbestos insulation used in houses?" Mom asked.

"I don't think it was used for insulation as much as ceiling tile and wrapping of heat pipes and boilers," the doctor said.

"It's the floating particles in the air you breathe that never absorb in or leave your lungs," Dad added.

"Has radiation been known to take care of this kind of cell?" asked Mom.

The doctor responded carefully, "Well, it certainly helps. We hope to be able to control it, but only time will tell."

"Now, after this radiation, what kind of test do you give to see if there's been an improvement?" Dad asked.

"Well, an ordinary X-ray would be helpful, and a CAT scan would be more helpful. It would be good to have a post-surgical CAT scan for a baseline," the doctor answered.

"There's a limit to the radiation they can give you," he went on. "I don't know if they plan to give you the limit the first six weeks or not. But if they do, that's pretty much what they can give you in that area. They can't go above 6,000-7,000 rads. If it cropped up someplace else in your body, then you could have more there, but in the same area, there's not a lot of tissue tolerance for more radiation."

"I see," said Dad as he took this in. "You might do more damage than good."

"That's right," replied the doctor. "The pathology report isn't back yet. They're doing electron microscopy to examine tissue. It takes about a week to prepare the tissue and make the picture on a micron microscope. They do additional studies to rule out other kinds of lung cancer, and they use special stains and do various immunologic tests to see if there are particular antigens or antibodies within the tissue. Pathologists do things to really nail down the diagnosis. We'll have that information. But, I don't think there's much question about what you have. It is mesothelioma."

Dad contemplated aloud, "When I retired and got out of the plant, I kept feeling better and better. But what happened thirty years ago is catching up with me."

The doctor added, "That's the thing with asbestos."

"Dad didn't smoke or have any symptoms," I said.

"This tumor's not related to smoking," the doctor explained. "However, if a person smokes and is exposed to asbestos, they have an extremely high risk of lung cancer. You do not have this. So, smoking is a factor in lung cancer, but it is not a factor in mesothelioma."

Dad stated further, "Now, lung cancer, if it hasn't spread, you can take out a little bit of lung and you're rid of it. But, you don't get this kind out as easily? Is that right?"

The doctor answered, "That's true. It's because it's spread. It's like taking a salt shaker and shaking it all over the chest. Yours is not that extensive, but it is still in a number of areas along the pleural surface. There's no way to get rid of every cell, unless it's totally localized. In that case, it would be a benign tumor. That's very rare, and I've actually only ever seen one case of it."

Dad asked about his pain, "Do you think, in a week or two, I'll feel better? It kind of gets me all over now."

"You can go ahead and take some pain pills," the doctor advised. Take extra-strength Tylenol during the day and stronger pain pills at night. They'll help you sleep."

The doctor concluded the appointment. "You've handled this exceedingly well. We'll say good-bye for now and I certainly wish you well. God bless you. It's been a pleasure to meet all of you."

Dad replied, "We feel comfortable with you."

"I'm glad it hasn't been all that bad of an experience," the doctor smiled as he shook our hands.

Dad had placed a strong trust in the doctor. He knew that the doctor, with his professional skill, had done everything possible during surgery. And with his parting statement, Dad had even looked for a bright side to the experience.

Chapter 13
Interlude and Return to Ohio

Even though I took notes and later transcribed them, the doctors had given revelations I didn't want to hear. Their tone with us had been conciliatory and hopeful, yet they had explained the unalterable facts of the disease.

Our sojourn to Seattle was ending. We had come, uncertain about Dad's cancer diagnosis. We would leave the Northwest with a specific name for the cancer and with apprehension about the future. The apprehension included meeting a new set of doctors in Sylvania and providing them with the necessary medical information.

My brother Dean phoned NIOSH (National Institute of Safety and Health), the federal agency which studies health and safety conditions in the workplace. He wanted to find out more about mesothelioma and other occupationally-caused diseases. From them, he received very technical information written in statistical and medical terms which were difficult for me to understand. None of the case studies suggested that there would be a promising outcome. Finding little information in medical books, I wondered if many persons were aware of the disease.

I reasoned that medical science knew little about mesothelioma since it wasn't like lung cancer or breast cancer with thousands of annual cases and proven treatments available. Perhaps there wasn't enough known about the disease to predict the outcome. That had to be the reason that articles I read recounted such grim figures or didn't list the disease at all. Part of it was my own denial.

I hoped Dad would be the patient who was different. His case had been detected at an early stage before any debilitating symptoms. He probably had several quality years left. All he had to do was make it through the treatments.

I began reading helpful books as I searched for answers. I looked for books about positive thinking during illness which were similar to the books by Dr. Bernie Siegel. With faith and knowledge, I thought Dad had a chance.

I decided my role would be a positive and encouraging one. Dad had always provided that for me. Even though I could never fully repay him, his recovery and comfort would be my primary concern.

When we returned to Ohio, we would be carrying a heavy load. Because of my proximity to my parents, I would be the offspring in charge. It would be my job to report Dad's progress to my brothers.

My brother Milan was not directly involved in the Seattle proceedings. His family lived in Philadelphia, and his young sons were still in school at the time of Dad's surgery. I sensed Milan's anguish in daily phone conversations, as it was hard enough to interpret Dad's progress while present. Usually when Milan talked to Dad, Dad was his typical upbeat self.

As I look back, there were things my father was never able to do after surgery. This occurred because of his pain and his weakened condition and because of the constant demand of dealing with cancer. Dad never again drove a car. He quit doing yard work. He stopped doing simple physical tasks he had once taken for granted. He never slept through the night free from pain. He constantly had to consider his diet and further treatments. And he was no longer available as a parent or grandparent in the same way. Granted, he was teaching us new things about dealing with illness. But given the cancer's progression, Dad's daily life changed rapidly.

I fondly remembered the times when he had been a strong parent. He had revealed to me that he was present in the delivery room when we children were born. Such a practice was uncommon at the time. He was the first one to hold us after birth. As an adult, this symbol of protection became significant to me.

I remembered a family reunion held at Indian Lake when I was about six years old. A cousin took us in his motorboat for a ride. As the boat's speed increased, the front end raised high in the air. I grabbed Dad's leg and held on tightly. As he gave me a gritted teeth smile, he never complained. When back on shore, he finally mentioned that his circulation had been in jeopardy during the ride!

Even though a monotone himself, Dad paid for lessons and musical concert tickets involving his family. These began with piano lessons and included band and orchestra programs from elementary school through college. Often, my parents sat in the front row at the concerts. Even when standing beside us in church, Dad's lack of pitch did not hinder his volume and enthusiasm for singing hymns.

Both my brothers played Little League baseball for the local Dodgers. I grew up thinking every family's summer schedule revolved around baseball games. My favorite parts were running under the bleachers and buying penny pretzels at the refreshment stand. I had faint interest in the game itself. But Dad and Mom knew each player and his batting average. Mom served as an official scorekeeper.

With heights of 6'4", my brothers also starred in high school basketball. Dad and Mom never missed a game, at home or away. A snake-like caravan enroute to the away games resembled the ones in the movie *Hoosiers*. Parents of the players carpooled. They counted on mingling on the way to the games, sitting and cheering at the games, and analyzing game highlights on the way home. After one especially exciting season, the other fathers decided to hang an Olympic-style medal around Dad's neck. They said Dad was the only one of the group who hadn't sworn at the referees all season!

While we were in college, Dad worked lots of overtime at the foundry. We three children managed to spend a total of eighteen years working on various degrees. During the same time, my mother, who had a two-year normal teaching degree, decided to complete her bachelor's degree. Dad helped pay tuition and co-sign numerous college loans. We never questioned our opportunity to go to college.

After Dad's surgery in Seattle, it was near the Fourth of July. Most kinds of fireworks are legal and openly for sale in Washington state. But what is the thrill of buying that kind of fireworks if there are more novel ones available on the Indian reservations? thought my teen-aged nephews. My brother and his wife left for a special anniversary weekend, and they designated us as house sitters. A list of chores for my nephews to accomplish was posted. Also, money was placed in an envelope for emergencies.

My nephews were nowhere to be seen for two days. We didn't know what to tell the girls who called for them. When they did return, they brought emergency pizzas, emergency fireworks, and an empty emergency envelope. They literally raced around mowing and doing chores before their parents' return. I reflected on growing up with my two brothers, and I decided times really hadn't changed that much.

Mary spoke with me before we left Seattle. She realized we would be facing a burden, and she said I shouldn't forget to do things for myself once in a while. I responded that my parents had power to cope with the future. Mary reminded me of support systems back home which had developed over a lifetime — relationships that would be important in the coming months. And even though there would be many miles between us, my brother and she were only a phone call away.

We arranged for our plane trip home during the busy summer season. Mary and I stood at the counter to get boarding passes as the computer noted our change in departure. No seats were available in coach, so the agent gave us three first-class seats. As my parents and I walked toward the gate, Dean wiped tears from his eyes.

If first-class seats seemed lucky, the opposite happened at our Chicago O'Hare transfer. The connecting flight was canceled, leaving an abandoned room of travelers. Both Mom and Dad were riding in wheelchairs as I tried to run between them with hand luggage. We were rerouted to another terminal and followed a trail of passengers. With the onslaught, that plane quickly filled, and we attempted two more flights before finally booking a plane at our original gate.

I had tried to explain Dad's health situation to airline employees. My tip money dwindled as assistants pushed the wheel chairs from gate to gate. When we finally boarded the Toledo-bound plane, the stewardess asked if anyone was willing to give up a seat. Dad said he wouldn't give his up for $10,000. It was late when we landed at the Toledo airport where my aunt and uncle had waited patiently to meet us.

Chapter 14
Meeting the Flower Hospital Oncologist

Our consultation with the oncologist at Sylvania's Flower Memorial Hospital took place on July 6, 1989. We delivered a shopping bag of X-rays, CAT scans, specimens, slides, and reports. We hoped the doctors understood what they all meant.

The oncology department was conveniently located on the ground floor, a short distance from the parking garage. Signs marked reserved spaces for oncology patients.

We met with the chairman of the Department of Oncology who had been in contact with the Seattle doctors, and he was anticipating our arrival. Wearing wire-rimmed glasses, the white-haired doctor appeared very studious, and his manner of speech was careful, yet warm. He listened politely as Dad repeated the history of his disease and treatment thus far.

Then, the doctor asked, "How are you feeling now?"

Dad replied he didn't feel so bad, but he was experiencing a deep pain which went all through his chest area. He added that the nerves frozen with liquid nitrogen felt different than the rest.

"Have you lost any weight?" the doctor asked.

"I don't weigh much over 150 now. I used to weigh 168-174," Dad answered.

"Have you had any change in your breathing since the surgery?" the doctor inquired.

"Not much," Dad responded. "They want me to cough and breathe deeply. It doesn't hurt me to breathe."

The doctor thought this was a good thing. Next, he asked Dad if he knew of any exposure to asbestos at the foundry.

Dad said, "I've come to the conclusion that back when I was hired in 1950, we had some hard boards on these vertical ovens that would stand the heat indefinitely. They were solid and had another mineral mixed in with them besides asbestos."

Then, the doctor examined Dad's chest area and back. He noted the tape burns which covered the incision. The incision itself was healing. The doctor explained that it had been a pretty miserable operation since the surgeon spread the ribs apart and cut through muscles. Dad said he was glad he hadn't lost a lobe of his lung.

"We brought you numerous materials plus the surgeon's report," Mom said. "Missing is the pathology report."

The doctor responded, "They're still waiting on special stains before they issue the report. Let me explain a little bit about the disease and treatment. This is a relatively rare tumor, although we're seeing it more commonly now than we did ten to fifteen years ago. It's one that's very difficult to treat. In fact, there's no known cure, because it tends to spread through the lining of the lung and coat it."

Dad asked, "It's mostly a disease of the lung, and doesn't go into the intestines?"

"On rare occasions, it can be seen there, too, but generally, it stays localized in the chest cavity," he answered. "There are cases reported in the abdominal cavity as well."

Dad inserted, "I was tested from head to toe, and they only found it in the right chest."

The doctor nodded and continued, "The treatment which seems to work best is to remove as much of the tumor nodule area as possible, and then give radiation to the lining of the lungs to kill off remaining cells. We've had experience here combining radiation with the chemotherapy Adriamycin, although one study didn't show Adriamycin as being beneficial. We do have experience with other cancers where giving platinum and radiation does seem to help. So it would be worthwhile to talk to the chemotherapist and see if he would be willing to combine chemotherapy with radiation treatments. The chemotherapy circulates in the body to kill cancer cells that may have spread to distant organs," the doctor concluded.

Concerned, Dad asked, "Would that hurt the rest of my system?"

"Well, the doses we're talking about are relatively low. It's unlikely to cause any significant reaction," the doctor replied. "Platinum does have side effects on the blood count, and it can be injurious to your kidneys. When you get it, you drink lots of fluids. I think chemotherapy can be safely done and be useful."

The doctor then explained radiation. "The radiation will be given to the entire lining of the right lung cavity to treat not only the nodules we know about, but the cells that are too small to see. Radiation will sterilize the disease and keep it from coming back, if possible. At the very least, it will delay it. Radiation would be given to the entire lung cavity for 4½ weeks, five days a week. Then, we would narrow down to the spot where the surgeon marked and treat that for another week and a half."

Dad asked, "Can you tell where the spots are?"

The doctor answered, "We use special X-rays for setting up your field. At the time we do markings for radiation, we would get CAT scans in several sections through your lungs to help plan radiation. We'll treat the entire lining of the lung while saving the center portion from the radiation."

The doctor then told about the effects of radiation including tiredness and burning of the skin. He said it's possible to have some nausea, but not likely. Toward the end of treatment, Dad would develop difficulty swallowing and feel like he had a lump in his throat because of swelling of the esophagus.

Dad asked, "As long as you can chew or swallow, you can eat most anything? But when you couldn't..."

"You'd have to eat more liquid foods," the doctor explained. "We have liquid foods we can give you if that becomes necessary. After treatment, these reactions die down. The sunburn changes to a tan. You will probably lose hair in the radiated area which may or may not grow back later. You may also have a dry, hacking cough caused by inflammation along the edges of the lung. In time, that goes away."

Dad wondered, "What percent of capacity would I have in the right lung when I'm done?"

"It would be hard to say," the doctor answered. "A rough guess is that you could do things at a walking pace without difficulty. When you walk up stairs or jog, you could be limited. Decreased capacity would develop over a period of months."

Dad wanted to know if that would be a temporary change. The doctor said that the change would be permanent. My father needed statistics. "Would I have only 50 percent on this side?"

"That would be a rough guess right now," the doctor agreed.

Dad spoke thoughtfully, "Some persons have one lung removed and get along pretty good. Does the other lung compensate and get a little bigger?"

The doctor explained that the lung can expand a little bit to the right side. Capacity wouldn't come back, and there would be scarring along the edges. If the tumor is not eradicated, in several years, it could start growing again and cause fluid to accumulate. Breathing would be compromised because of pressure on the lung to collapse it. With that alternative, the doctor felt it was worthwhile to sacrifice some of the lung to prevent that from happening.

"It'll be a little new for me," Dad stated.

"He's been the strong one at our house," Mom said.

"Well, I'm going to help him get through this," the doctor promised.

Dad asked, "For tumor control, this is pretty new, isn't it?"

"Well, actually, this kind of treatment has been going on for about six to eight years for mesothelioma," the doctor responded. Mom explained that Dean had sent papers with names of the Seattle doctors who could be contacted for further information. Dad asked if one doctor could read another doctor's handwriting. The oncologist laughed and said it took a lot of practice.

I asked, "Do you mostly do these steps for treatment now, and then later on, try some other treatment?"

The doctor said, "Well, I hope this is successful. But if the disease reoccurs, then we might have to consider either some additional radiation or different chemotherapy."

"The Seattle surgeon mentioned using interferon," I stated.

"That's a new drug," the doctor replied, "without much known benefit for the disease, but I guess it's being worked on. Some of the stronger drugs are the better agents right now."

He continued, "I'll make an appointment with the chemotherapy doctor and also make one for you to receive the markings for radiation." The doctor made note of educational offerings including sessions called I Can Cope, sponsored by the Cancer Society, and monthly programs at Flower.

The doctor reassured Dad that he was healed and ready to begin radiation. We then watched a video about what to expect during radiation. We absorbed information about the next leg of our journey on this roller coaster ride.

Chapter 15
Issuing the Results

The official pathology report, which included tests done on surgery specimens, arrived in Ohio in early July. The report was written on July 1, 1989, by a doctor at the Laboratory of Pathology at Seattle. Specimens were also tested at the Diagnostic Specialties Laboratory in Bremerton, Washington. The results covered extensive tests on six specimens, since only a preliminary observation of them had been done the day of surgery.

The lab received the specimens in six parts, labeled A-F. Operating room consultants had noted that the nodular mass from the pleural wall showed a spindle cell neoplasm suggestive of mesothelioma. Further testing in the lab had to be done to verify the final diagnosis. Before the pathology report was received, one could imagine that the diagnosis was possibly some other form of cancer, perhaps a treatable kind.

The official pathology report included:

Section A: Nodular mass from parietal pleura (outer wall of membrane around the lung)

The nodular mass from the upper right pleura was egg-shaped and had a tan-white, fibrous appearance. The mass was a malignant spindle cell neoplasm with transparent epithelial (outer) cells. The cancer cells were in various stages of growth with prominent and multiple nucleoli and indistinct cell borders. Necrosis, or death of tissue, was not a feature.

Sections C and E: Pleural Tissue

Sizes of the pleural tissue ranged from two to twelve cm long. Pleural tissue over the right lower lobe was a plaque of tan-pink, firm cancerous tissue. Pleural tissue from the right upper lobe had been attached to the lung. A cross-section revealed largely benign lung tissue, partly surrounded by adherent tumor tissue.

The cancer cells had an oval to spindle-shaped nucleus. Patchy collections of lymphocytes (white blood cells) were noted along the edge of the pleura. The underlying lining showed fibrosis between tissues, anthracotic (dust) deposits, acute damage to air sacs, collections of histiocytes (immune system cells in tissue), and inflammatory cells with dust deposits.

Section D: Diaphragm

Section D was a biopsy of the diaphragm. The specimen was a flat portion of tan-white, fibrous neoplastic tissue which measured 3 by 2 by .2 cm. After surgery, the doctor had mentioned extensive cancer nodules on the diaphragm.

Sections B and F: Segments of fifth and sixth ribs

Section B had been part of the fifth and sixth rib bones that were removed in order to make surgery possible. Section F also included part of a rib and some pleura from the posterior. There was no evidence of metastatic tumor in the bones.

Asbestos digestion analysis

Section A, the malignant mesothelioma invading the lung tissue, was submitted to the lab for further testing. A test was done to determine the number of asbestos bodies present in the specimen as compared to the general population. The pathologist used a special technique and machine to separate the asbestos fibers from the tissue.

A five gram sample of lung tissue was cut into small pieces and completely digested in commercial bleach. Then, the bleach was carefully decanted, which means the liquid was poured off. Next, the sediment at the bottom of the container was extracted, or drawn out, with equal volumes of chloroform and 50% ethyl alcohol.

The above solution was transferred to a test tube, shaken vigorously, and centrifuged, or rotated, at 1200 rpm for ten minutes. After removal of as much material containing carbon as possible, the solution was recentrifuged. The sediment at the bottom of the test tube was extracted in 95% alcohol and passed through a Millipore filter of .5 micrometer diameter pore size. Asbestos bodies on the filter were then counted.

Asbestos count study

The results of the asbestos count were as follows. The sample lung tissue demonstrated 970 ferruginous (containing iron) bodies per gram of wet lung tissue. Most of these bodies appeared to have cores of translucent yellow-white material consistent with asbestos or asbestos bodies. A few had black cores which raised the possibility of an additional non-asbestos ferruginous body as well.

The pathologist at the Diagnostic Specialties Laboratory concluded that the number of asbestos bodies in the sample was significantly elevated over the numbers seen in the general urban population without a history of occupational exposure to asbestos. And this finding, he wrote, would indicate that this patient's mesothelioma was caused by asbestos.

I hadn't known that it was possible to have lungs surrounded by asbestos fibers. The fibers could be as permanent in the human body as anywhere else, I supposed. The body could not absorb them or break them down. Was that why asbestos was hailed as the miracle mineral in the first place — because of its indestructibility? How could my father have been exposed to asbestos so long ago and just now be paying the price? How were the asbestos manufacturers able to produce such a physically harmful product for so long?

Chapter 16
Surviving from Treatment to Treatment

The results of the pathology report, along with the surgical report, sounded ominous to me. This kind of cancer really happens. The outlook seemed grim. How were we going to get through this ordeal? What quality of life would Dad have and for how long? The surgeon's comments about time limits and pain control were constantly echoing in my ears.

During the first few weeks at home, I tried to broach the subject of Dad's prognosis. Even though outwardly, Dad was recuperating well, I wanted others to share the inward grief and uncertainties. With most persons, I would carry on so Dad's daily life was as normal as possible. But, significant persons should be aware of the eventual outcome.

At an informal meeting, I mentioned the prognosis to our minister. I hesitated to set a time limit because I didn't want such an actuality. Each case is different, I said, and everything possible would be done in hopes of prolonging Dad's life. However, it was multiple tumor involvement we were dealing with.

Our minister was a young woman in her first pastorate. She had called us periodically in Seattle. Dad had respected her and they worked closely since Dad served the church as treasurer. I wondered if she understood our dilemma. Did she know what it was like to be losing a parent? Could she offer solace and words of encouragement when the going got rough? Would Dad be able to share his deepest concerns with her? Because Dad appeared so energetic, it was hard to convey my message.

Mom hesitated to tell her brother and his wife about Dad's condition. I thought they should know that we definitely had a battle, and yet we were not giving up hope. When I talked to them, I could barely get the words out. They reacted with shock and concern for how my mother would cope.

A close friend of mine also had a relative who had worked at

General Motors. He had died of cancer two years before. Doctors had not diagnosed his specific condition and had been treating his pneumonia symptoms. My friend related what her family had experienced including how debilitated the man became.

I hoped my friend would now empathize with me. I explained what we thought had caused my father's condition. I said that, so far, no one had ever been cured of this kind of cancer. I am grateful for her positive response to me that day. She replied that maybe my father would be the first one cured, that he could be the exception. I had needed to hear that there was still hope. Such an attitude is necessary before starting the cycle of radiation treatments.

Four days after we met with the oncologist, Dad went for a baseline X-ray and for special X-rays to simulate, or set up, the plan for radiation. The therapist used black and red markers to outline places on my Dad's chest, neck, and back where the radiotherapy would be directed. Pinpointing exact locations with the tattoo dots was important because this would become an initial map to use. Later, metal shields of lead would be cut in the shape surrounding the treatment areas to protect normal tissue. Dad was told not to wash the marked places and to have Mom re-mark them if they wore off.

Prior to radiation, a prospective patient signs a permission form which acknowledges plans for treatment. The form warns that such treatment can indirectly cause permanent damage to surrounding tissues and organs such as the heart, lungs, and esophagus. Dad read and signed the form. He was ready to start daily treatments to prolong his life and, hopefully, stunt the tumors.

Dad's dosages of radiation would be computed mathematically as his charts were studied. Since some of the radiation would penetrate clear through, and other radiation would go only to a certain depth, amounts had to be strictly adhered to. Dad would receive radiation from two different machines in two different rooms.

On the day of the markings, we also met with the chemotherapy doctor. First, a young resident questioned Dad about his entire medical history, which gave us doubts about whether or not the doctors had studied his medical records. This added to our anxiety until the regular doctor came in.

The chemotherapy specialist, originally from Pakistan, spoke hurriedly, but knowledgeably. He said he would search for a protocol which fit Dad. Some of the protocols had age limits because of toxicity. He decided he would discuss the possibilities with the oncology staff.

Dad asked what effect the chemo would have on him. The doctor replied that the platinum has side effects on the kidneys. Other effects could be in the form of skin reactions or lowered blood counts. Loss of body hair would not be a concern. There might be nausea and vomiting. Dad proudly stated that he hadn't thrown up in fifty years.

When asked about reduced lung capacity, the doctor said there would be fibrosis, or scarring, of the air sacs in the lungs. Dad again realized that he would have to sacrifice some breathing capacity in order to fight the cancer cells.

Dad wanted to know if his breathing would be painful after reduced capacity. The doctor responded that the tumors are more likely to cause pain than the treatments. Since the tumors involve sensitive structures, there can be pain in the nerves.

The chemotherapist didn't like to dwell on the fact, but he said that whatever treatment Dad got, it wouldn't be a curative one. It could not erase the disease or get rid of it forever. Dad wondered what to do when the cells came back. The doctor said there are different ways to deal with it, but we should take one step at a time.

Dad also wondered if the cancer was likely to break out in the other lung. The doctor responded that there were no guarantees. The cancer could go elsewhere, but since it wasn't in the other lung, that factor was a good thing.

For the daily treatment schedule, I marked the days on my calendar. Many persons offered help, but this didn't always include a whole day of traveling and waiting for medical appointments. Some didn't understand that it was a daily 130-mile round trip, not a weekly one. Regardless of who drove, Mom planned to go every day.

In addition to the radiation treatment, Dad met with the oncologist early in the week and with the counselor on Fridays. This added more hours to the day. If radiotherapy patients were behind schedule, we got delayed. Since Dad used two machines, he sometimes waited for one or the other.

Weekly chemotherapy was added to the radiation about the third week of treatment. As Dad sat in a reclining chair, platinum dripped from an IV into his veins. Before receiving platinum, Dad was given fluids and anti-nausea medication intravenously. The entire process, supervised by an Oncology Certified Nurse, or OCN-RN, required four hours minimum. We kept Dad company in the chemo room. We were told that side effects vary, and they do not necessarily indicate the chemotherapy's effectiveness.

On certain days, Dad was scheduled for X-rays and had to be at the hospital earlier. Mom and I made the trip with Dad almost every day with an occasional day of rest. Unfortunately, Dad could never take a day off. Volunteers from church drove, and my uncle told Mom to stay home when he took Dad. Mom used these days off to sort through medical bills which arrived from Seattle in bundles.

At our appointments with doctors, we asked questions about diet, energy levels, activities Dad could do, and effects of radiation. We would take a list of questions. Group participation helped us remember what the doctor had said and helped us understand and discuss the treatment. When Mom asked one doctor if he had ever had a patient's family with so many questions, he responded that we were definitely among his top ten.

The oncology center was only one story high and was located between the medical center and the hospital. Its rooms had unusual geometric shapes. The radiation area had a skylight and several small rooms which opened into a central waiting room.

Positioned along one wall, the radiation therapy technologists viewed their monitor screens. A ledge above them held equipment, and a higher shelf held patient files and the framed certificates of the technologists. The technologists, all women, donned white jackets. A man occasionally came by to check the operation of the machines.

The two radiation rooms in use had wide, thick doors and warning signs posted near them. An attending technologist announced a patient's name. Once inside the small room, she helped the patient get undressed and situated under the machine. Then, she exited the room and operated the machine by looking at the patient on a screen and pushing appropriate buttons while keeping verbal contact on an intercom. When the radiation machine was operating, a white light appeared above the closed door. To the patient lying under it, the machine sounded like a vacuum cleaner. The actual dosage required only one to five minutes. Dad received treatment in several spots.

Radiation uses a machine which generates a high energy beam in brief, high level doses. The beam destroys cancer cells by penetrating body tissue. One kind of machine, for external therapy, treats cancer near the skin's surface. Another machine treats cancer deep in the body. Radiation, or radiotherapy, is second only to surgery as the most common form of cancer treatment. The amount of radiation depends on the size, location, and the cell type of the tumor.

In the case of advanced disease, radiation may not be a curative thing. We learned that radiation can assist in relieving symptoms and the pain, and it can improve the quality of a patient's life. Radiation itself is painless. Persons lose weight during radiation because of poor appetite and difficulty in chewing and swallowing. Patients also have trouble maintaining energy levels and avoiding infections. Good cells as well as cancer cells lose their ability to grow and divide after radiotherapy. Normal cells recover more rapidly, especially during weekend breaks from treatments.

In the waiting area, all the patients receiving radiotherapy had one thing in common. They had cancer. I remember one lady who drove herself to treatments because she had no one to assist her. Another lady was having a second series of radiation for a recurring breast cancer. One man could only speak through a special microphone which he held under his chin. He was a repeat radiation patient, having lost his voice box to surgery. Another man had cancer in his jaw, and one could readily see the darkened radiation spot near his throat. Another woman said she and her husband both had cancer. Patients were all ages, though not many children came. Several nuns, dressed in modified black habits, received radiation. Some patients came in wheelchairs. Others arrived in hospital beds, presumably pushed from their rooms. Almost all the patients, in the midst of treatments, were rail thin because of the continuous assault on their bodies.

Twice during his treatments, Dad experienced fainting spells. After chemotherapy was added to the radiation, one became concerned about numbers. By then, we were keeping track of white blood counts, red blood counts, and platelet counts. A low white count made Dad susceptible to infection. A low red count indicated anemia. Too few platelets caused bruises to the skin and lack of blood clotting. We became greatly concerned about numbers, especially midweek after chemo. If the counts were too low, Dad couldn't tolerate further treatments until the counts began to rise.

Dad's fainting spells had been caused by a dip in blood pressure, a side effect of treatment. The nurses had noticed Dad's weakness and had come to our rescue with a wheelchair. They assured Dad that this was common. The doctor also provided reassurance.

The daily trip to Sylvania provided us time to be together. We felt we were doing something constructive about the cancer. We enjoyed the rides, often singing and listening to humorous tapes.

We stopped along the highway at summer vegetable markets and ice cream drive-ins. We discovered variations in routes to the hospital. Dad sat in the back seat with a pillow and blanket. Mom and I took turns driving. We found the trips a good outlet. Toward the end, we definitely needed two persons, one to drive and one to take care of Dad.

There was no opportunity to plan other types of activity. Scratch off normal routines for a cancer patient. The patient is consumed with travel to treatments and worry about his progress. No clear-cut answers are provided. From the first post-surgical X-ray, doctors told us that there had been no change. Those words are difficult to interpret.

We never did make it to a cancer education session. I had good intentions and even wrote the dates on my calendar. Somehow, time always ran out. However, we read several helpful books and tried to keep our outlook positive.

By the time treatments were ending, I wanted to be a thousand miles away or wherever the daily routine involved a more light-hearted activity. Reacting to a flight response, I went on a mini-vacation in late August by myself. I returned in time to drive Dad to his final treatment. Would treatments really soon be over?

I thought Dad had gotten through the radiation fairly well. He was still physically active. Chemo usually knocked him out for a day, and then he would bounce back. He went for walks and had not lost any breathing capacity. Mom and Dad even scheduled a bus trip to Nashville with the county retired teachers.

We didn't know what to expect next. Radiation works in the system a long time after actual treatments stop. Dad looked like a whipped puppy. He could hardly get up from a chair. His face was sunken, and he lost more weight. He barely swallowed liquids and would spend two to three hours eating a bowl of lukewarm soup. Since he was determined not to lose additional weight, we bought all liquid nutrients for him.

Even worse, the radiated areas turned raw and red. When removing his shirt, Dad would also remove a layer of skin which oozed bloody pus .

Gradually, Dad's strength returned. We used this encouraging sign to the best advantage. We talked about how much better Dad would feel in another week. We dangled the upcoming Nashville trip before him. And Dad looked forward to visits from both his sons.

In the fall, Dad was re-elected to a new three-year term as the church's treasurer. Doing this job took many hours of his time.

We thought this was a way for him to remain active and useful when some of his other activities had been restricted. This helped us consider the future as possibly an ongoing trail ahead.

Chapter 17
Seeking Quality of Living

All during the summer, we encouraged Dad to keep a positive frame of mind. Such an outlook was not foreign to Dad. Many of the books I encountered about cancer and coping with illness stressed this concept. I read them for my own survival as well as for Dad's benefit. Given the usual progression of the disease, what did we have to lose by thinking good thoughts?

I scoured bookstores for books and tapes on cancer. I skimmed medical books to find out about asbestos diseases, looking for more encouraging statistics. I read about new cancer treatments, perhaps ones that offered more promise of a cure. This burdened me because the answer was always going to be in the next book I found.

Instead of receiving understanding from others, I felt others were overly optimistic. Since the cure rate is now nearly fifty percent, cancer is no longer a feared, hushed word. Many treatments are used successfully. A cancer patient is at least expected to go into an extended remission. Besides, Dad was walking around looking fairly healthy.

Well meaning acquaintances had asked the repetitive question immediately after surgery. "Did they get all the cancer out?" I carefully answered that Dad had a kind of cancer in which removal of all the tumors was impossible. People would often change the subject, and some even repeated the question as if re-asking would improve the response.

At the hospital, the oncology staff was especially sensitive to the psychological needs of cancer patients. Their manner was sympathetic and helpful, and they concerned themselves with the family members as well. At times, I needed their support and understanding as much as Dad.

The receptionists were forthright and efficient. They called each patient by name. They answered special concerns, directed us to the right location, and scheduled the next needed test.

Author and researcher, Norman Cousins, had recently spoken at a convention in Washington, D.C. He introduced his newest book, *Head First, the Biology of Hope,* regarding a patient's positive mental attitude having a favorable impact upon disease. I had listened to his theories. Mr. Cousins, an adjunct professor at the UCLA School of Medicine, evolved his theory from personal experience. After receiving a poor prognosis for a connective tissue disease, Cousins reversed the situation by his own method of cure. He used a wide range of positive emotions to his body's advantage. Currently, he is involved in research on the therapeutic value of positive emotions.

Since negative emotions have been accepted as harmful to human health, why couldn't positive emotions favorably influence the immune system? he asked. The brain, as part of the nervous system, produces glandular secretions throughout the body. Therefore, a person's mental state could play a significant role in the biochemical balance of the body. Cousins doesn't consider this approach a denial of the illness, but an active participation in using the body's own resources to combat the illness (Cousins, 1989, 86-87). I later bought Cousin's book for Dad to read.

Because of possible litigations, I had to agree that doctors give patients the worst possible scenarios of what could happen with their diseases. Doctors don't promise how anything is going to work. I learned that they just don't know. Doctors describe the worst, perhaps not considering the power of positive suggestion or the fighting spirit the patient may bring with him.

A source of easygoing entertainment we used was Garrison Keillor audio tapes. We listened to Keillor's homespun tales of life in the mythical town of Lake Wobegon. Keillor's witty humor and soothing voice capture universal stories of human nature. I often thought about letting Mr. Keillor know how much we enjoyed his storytelling and singing while enroute to cancer treatments.

I was knowledgeable about the typical reactions persons normally experience in a life-threatening crisis. These traits are discussed in the book, *I Can Cope — Staying Healthy with Cancer* by Judi Johnson and Linda Klein. The traits include disbelief, anger, denial, depression, and uncertainty, not necessarily in that order. These reactions apply to both the patient and to members of his family. Everyone is on board for the roller coaster ride.

One usually thinks that cancer is a disease that happens to someone else. Disbelief is a shield against the shocking reality that now the unimagined includes your loved one and you.

Anger can take many forms. It doesn't always involve shouting or open hostility. Sometimes, it includes questions such as "Why is this happening?" or "Why wasn't it diagnosed sooner?" Dad had thought that the doctors at the foundry's annual chest X-ray screening had never noticed any problems with his lungs. At other times, anger comes during the frustrating delay of waiting for answers. While you thought your parent was in good health, the insidious asbestos fibers were inside him wreaking havoc. After his years of hard work and clean living, one considers how undeserved the diagnosis is.

Denial helps one continue to function in everyday life. After all, there is only so much that a person can absorb at once. Denial gives one time to adjust to a major change in daily focus. In our case, the medical reports with a definitive diagnosis and the pressing need to plan treatments made continued denial useless.

One can waver in and out of depression during the span of the illness. There is loss of control over daily activities. A robust member of the family is suddenly viewed as vulnerable. One pictures the cancer cells multiplying wildly and traveling from organ to organ. Doctors don't even know where the cancer cells are, and there's no way to tell. One tries to regain control by becoming informed and involved in the treatment process and focusing on hopeful signs.

The uncertainty and fear is that cancer is a diminishing countdown. One learns to take single steps. Each day, there are questions about what is happening. One feels pressure to make the right choices. One wonders about the pain levels. One considers if the patient feels support from others. And there is the ultimate fear of facing the funeral of a parent and the emotions accompanying it. There is the anxiety that the next generation in line is one's own.

Besides general reading, I read about this particular disease. I wondered why I had never heard about it before and why so little was known. I wondered why an effective treatment had not been found. I began to understand why critically ill patients seek unconventional cures. If they could just find one that works, their search would be worthwhile.

I had previously read theories about the cancer personality. I even applied these theories to cancer victims I knew. The puzzle of their traits and cancer never quite fit together. I believe the development of personality is a complicated process, and life experiences are extensive and varied. It didn't seem that the myriad of persons getting cancer all had similar traits. If they did, then perhaps our society has a problem with how persons are allowed to express themselves.

Since my Dad's cancer was proven to be carcinogenic, I didn't know if the theory of a self-denying personality was accurate. Dad's zest for retirement certainly wasn't repressive nor was he an overly conforming individual. In fact, he seemed rather unique to me. He participated in personally meaningful activities and enjoyed his hobbies. Dad was positive toward others, and he reacted by giving humorous comments. I read about persons who put others first as more likely candidates for cancer. Such reading did inspire nagging doubts.

The challenge of facing illness gives the patient new purpose. Unimportant trivialities fall by the wayside. Illness is a realization that one's body is mortal and that time among family and friends is indeed precious. It provides a period to reassess one's life and evaluate past goals and future purpose. Illness is an opportunity to decide how one will face his most extraordinary challenge.

I found Dr. Bernie Siegel's insights, written in his two best-sellers, especially applicable to a cancer patient's struggle. From experience, he knew that a cancer patient is searching for hope and meaning from his illness. I thank Dr. Siegel for his words of wisdom, as his second book appeared in bookstores simultaneously with Dad's cancer diagnosis and surgery. His text provided a road map in what first seemed like an obstacle course.

Dr. Siegel espoused that patients are not helpless and that in the most desperate circumstances, the patient's outlook can bring peace of mind and sometimes lead to an unexpected cure (Siegel, 1989, 242). Like Cousins, he was saying that a cancer victim can beneficially reignite his own immune system.

Dr. Siegel's patients express themselves through drawings which he skillfully studies. Then, he interprets the symbols and what they reveal. He also promotes meditation and imaging. He says that a patient can visualize anything from a successful surgical outcome to the capture and annihilation of cancer cells by radiation.

I was interested in these positive visualizations much more than Dad. He probably felt I was pushing them on him. When Dad didn't have time to read the books, I purchased tapes for him. Dad did read some books on coping with cancer, but he never got very excited about the imaging meditation.

During the radiation treatments, the hospital counselor/chaplain informed us that Bernie Siegel would be leading a workshop at a nearby college. I considered this a great opportunity to hear

Siegel's philosophy about exceptional cancer patients firsthand, and we promptly signed up.

When October came, Dad had been recuperating for about a month and a half. The auditorium was nearly packed for the lecture. Many healthcare workers were in the audience. We anticipated an evening of insight about how each patient has healing potential within himself.

Dr. Siegel personified the caring, loving, and informed professional that his books portrayed. I would have paid just to hear his comforting voice and the quality of hope he conveyed. On a large screen, he showed drawings done by his patients. He could interpret a patient's condition and outlook by analyzing the pictures. I found it a curious phenomenon. Dad had trouble sitting comfortably, but he thoughtfully absorbed these ideas.

Since our local church planned to sponsor a program on caregiving, my mother inquired at Flower Hospital about possible seminars. She discovered that the hospital chaplain, the Reverend James Flinchbaugh, was an experienced workshop leader and would come to Bryan as part of the hospital's outreach. He often conducted sessions on dealing with the terminally ill and the grief process.

Arrangements were made for two sessions to be held midwinter on Sunday afternoons. Rev. Flinchbaugh suggested that sessions be limited to about thirty participants for an effective program. Mom hoped that by the time of the seminar, Dad and other local cancer patients would be able to share their experiences. But, by the first session, Dad was hospitalized in Flower with pneumonia.

Rev. Flinchbaugh was a Methodist minister who now served as chaplain at Flower Hospital. The hospital required cancer patients to meet with him at least once during treatments and on a continuing basis as needed. Rev. Flinchbaugh also worked with other patients and counseled family members who were dealing with the circumstances of illness. His office was at the hospital's main entrance across from the chapel. But more often than not, Rev. Flinchbaugh worked elsewhere in the hospital. He wore a beeper on his arm, and like some physicians, he was on call twenty-four hours a day.

Rev. Flinchbaugh divided the seminar into three parts: grief ministries, understanding needs of the elderly, and helping cancer patients. Through the use of group discussion, video programs, handouts, and lectures, Rev. Flinchbaugh ably conducted the sessions.

Regarding grief, he stressed that a loss causes shock and numbness the first weeks, and the loving presence of family and friends is needed. Experiencing the pain fully and deeply can take as long as a year. The three most common feelings of grief are guilt, anger, and fear. Unless these feelings are released, healing can be blocked. The grieving person needs to accept the agonizing reality of the loss until it no longer holds power over him. Many of these ideas were in a video about grief narrated by Howard Clinebell.

The seminar stressed helpful things which can be done to help grieving persons. By working together, the seminar participants listed these ideas:

HELPING GRIEVING PERSONS

1. Go to them and tell them, "I care."
2. Offer your presence and support.
3. Listen confidentially.
4. Assure them, "I'll be with you," and touch them.
5. Give them your time.
6. Avoid giving platitudes or saying, "I know how you feel."
7. Don't burden them with trivial business.
8. Send them cards.
9. Offer transportation to places.
10. Offer spiritual support through intercessory prayer.

The second part of the seminar included understanding the needs of older persons, especially if they are confined. There is the need to feel loved and wanted, the need to be socially involved, the need to feel useful, and the need for positive affirmation. All persons have these needs, but they are strongly felt by the elderly.

The part of the workshop dealing with cancer patients affected me the most. Even though Dad couldn't participate, there were several cancer patients present. Hints were given for family and friends, suggestions were given for visiting the sick, and ideas were discussed for the cancer patient himself. A synopsis of these three areas follows.

HINTS FOR FAMILY AND FRIENDS OF CANCER PATIENTS

1. Cook a dinner and deliver it in a disposable container.
2. Call before you visit and make the visit brief.
3. Offer to do a specific job or run an errand.
4. Allow the patient to feel emotions and express yours.
5. Let the patient express fears.
6. Talk about normal, everyday activities.

7. Offer to spend an evening visiting or watching television.
8. Share humorous anecdotes.
9. Tell the patient how great he looks by finding some positive features about him.
10. Talk about the future.

HOW TO VISIT A CANCER PATIENT

1. Make frequent, short visits.
2. Refrain from talk about your own or other cases of illness.
3. Be natural and cheerful.
4. Stay away if you yourself are carrying infections.
5. Give undivided attention, but avoid being inquisitive.
6. Be positive about the health care that is taking place.

IDEAS FOR THE CANCER PATIENT

The cancer patient should realize that his attitude keeps hope alive. Family members may have their own coping problems. Communication can be open and not be a pretense that everything is okay. Questions about the disease should be directed to the doctor who should also be told about any changes in the patient's physical condition. The patient should find reasons to live and express love to others. If arrangements for insurance policies, future health care measures, and funerals can be discussed beforehand, this eases stress on the family and considers the input of the patient.

The seminar was enlightening and in agreement with other ideas I read on caregiving. In my father's absence, I spoke briefly to the group. I mentioned how dealing with cancer is a family affair. I brought up the difficulty of witnessing a loved one's suffering and the uncertainties of the disease.

Our research in positive thinking was making a difference. Most of the time, Dad was cheerful. He showed exceptional courage in tolerating various treatments. He spoke about the future and things he wanted to accomplish. Because of Dad's bright attitude, some acquaintances had not realized the extent of his illness. The philosophy of making use of positive emotions was actually working for us.

Chapter 18
On Being Exposed Occupationally

During daily treatments at the hospital, I met a woman who was undergoing radiation for breast cancer. In conversation, I discovered that her husband was suffering from asbestosis. Previously employed in the Toledo area, he now had reduced breathing capacity and had filed a workman's compensation claim through an area attorney. She had collected news articles about asbestos and information on workman's compensation claims. When I expressed interest, she offered to bring materials with her the next day. Since I was also gathering information, I gratefully accepted her input.

In the second news section of the Toledo paper, I noticed a news item about an asbestos lawsuit in a neighboring county. Twenty-eight companies which handle asbestos and related products were named in the wrongful-death suit. The suit was filed by the widow of a man who had worked in a foundry for twenty-nine years. As I read, I wondered what foundry it might be. Since the lawsuit was a public record, I went to their courthouse to read a copy of the suit.

The man had worked in a core room where he had been a supervisor. It was not the same foundry where my father had worked. The suit stated, in part, that the victim's premature death from asbestosis and silicosis had been directly caused by the negligence of the listed companies. The companies had ignored scientific data which specifically stated that asbestos and related products were harmful and deadly to workers who came in contact with it.

In a nutshell, the suit stated further that the named defendants failed to advise the victim of the dangerous characteristics of asbestos, failed to provide knowledge of proper attire, and failed to place warnings on containers. The defendants also failed to publish, adopt, and enforce a safety plan for using the products, and they failed to provide directions for the handlers of the materials. To the general public, the defendants had implied that their materials were safe, marketable, and fit for use, and that the products contained no latent defects. In actuality, the materials were none of these things.

The victim suffered serious, permanent bodily injuries and death as a direct result of his reliance on said warranties. He had been frequently subjected to the inhalation of asbestos and silica dust which permeated the premises where he worked. He suffered multiple physical trauma, conscious pain and suffering, and incurred medical and hospital expenses. Upon his death, the family members lost such things as companionship, protection, advice, care and counsel, and they suffered mental anguish.

Listed at the bottom of the document was the name of a lawyer associated with a law firm in Holland, a Toledo suburb. Under his firm's name was a law firm in Barnwell, South Carolina. I shared these findings with my brother in Seattle. As a result, Dean called the Holland lawyer, Mr. Charles Contrada, to inquire about his experience with cases related to asbestos. We scheduled an informal meeting with Mr. Contrada to discuss Dad's situation and to decide if Dad wanted to consider a suit of his own.

At the Holland law firm, we were ushered into Mr. Contrada's office for the consultation. Mr. Contrada, an attorney for eleven years, specializes in injury cases which include asbestos. We had come directly from the hospital, and Dad was tired. Mr. Contrada asked how Dad was doing.

Dad replied, "I'm almost done with my radiation. I had chemotherapy, too. That's tough and it makes you more tired and washed out all the time. My back and chest cavity are nearly as sore as the week after the operation. I can stand a little bit of activity, though."

I added, "Maybe now, he'll have a little time to recuperate."

In our discussion, we found that there were no current comparable lawsuits filed by workers from Central Foundry in Defiance. Mr. Contrada remembered talking with my brother. Dean had also contacted the law firm in South Carolina which answers difficult questions about asbestos on a national level. Mr. Contrada said that the two law firms coordinate their work. In December of 1988, an asbestos case, filed in Lucas County, was brought to successful conclusion by Mr. Contrada. Consequently, Toledo area cases are referred to him.

Dad proceeded to explain his medical history and the disease and treatment for his mesothelioma. He said chest X-rays were given to the employees once a year at the health screening on the premises of Central Foundry. At the time of his retirement, he also had an X-ray in Bryan. He thought it showed no abnormalities. Dad stated he had no prior health problems.

Mr. Contrada said that the latency period for mesothelioma was typically fifteen to twenty years, and sometimes thirty years after initial exposure. Dr. Irving Selikoff from Mount Sinai Hospital in New York, which specializes in asbestos disease research, said that the chrysotile fiber, a type of asbestos, can cause mesothelioma. This assertion had previously been refuted. Mr. Contrada said that he believes that the type of asbestos fiber has nothing to do with the cause of mesothelioma and that you can get it from any kind of asbestos. And the extent of exposure which produces disease is currently not known.

"Proof in law and proof in medicine are two different things," Mr. Contrada continued. "Proof in law has more to do with probabilities. It is known that about 80 percent of mesotheliomas are caused by asbestos and that the only known cause of mesothelioma is asbestos exposure." He added that in about 20 percent of cases, a definite asbestos exposure cannot be pinpointed.

I wondered if, in that 20 percent, the exposure was from a more indirect cause, such as living near a factory which used asbestos or being exposed in public buildings which contained asbestos in their construction. Mr. Contrada said that the fact Dad had worked at the same job for over thirty years would make a big difference in tying down asbestos companies which provided materials.

Mr. Contrada explained that there are two issues in filing a claim in Ohio. One is to prove exposure to a certain asbestos product in which the identity of the manufacturer can be found. The product can be raw asbestos or asbestos in any other form. To help persons remember products, the law firm had a book with pictures of asbestos products used widely in the fifties and sixties. Product identification can be proven with live testimony by persons who remember or it can be proven by documents such as purchase records for which legal access can be gained. The local UAW may also have information. The second issue in Ohio is to prove medically that the disease process was related to or caused by asbestos. Dad certainly had decisive medical proof for that part, I concluded.

Mr. Contrada described how Dr. Irving Selikoff had blown the whistle on asbestos manufacturers. In 1964, he presented his studies on workers exposed to asbestos. He gave his message in New York at the international "Conference on the Biological

Effects of Asbestos," which was sponsored by the New York Academy of Sciences. Dr. Selikoff furnished irrefutable evidence that industrial exposure to asbestos was extremely hazardous. This disclosure brought changes in how health care professionals viewed asbestos exposure.

As early as the 1930s, producers who manufactured and processed asbestos knew their product caused lung problems. By the 1940s, they also knew that exposure to asbestos caused lung cancer. Mr. Contrada contended that the manufacturers covered up that information in order to market a profitable product. There are documents from Johns-Manville, a major marketer of asbestos, that say it would be cheaper to fight widows in workman's compensation cases than to tell employees to wear respirators which suggest that asbestos products are harmful. Dr. Selikoff believes that asbestos-caused diseases and lawsuits resulting from them will continue to increase through the year 2010, partly because of the latency period of the disease. After that, he believes that cases will decline because of more recent government-enforced cutbacks in the use of asbestos.

Dad told about his work in the core room at the foundry where engine cores were made from a sand formula. He said his plant made castings for engine blocks, both differential housing and transmission housing — anything that was a poured gray-iron casting. The castings were made in the rough and then sent to the Lansing, Michigan, plant to be honed out as cylinders and tapped for spark plugs. Over the years, the method of making the cores has changed, but the product has stayed the same. Before 1960, the cores were made from an oil and sand mixture. After that, the cores were made more quickly using the "hot box" method. A sand formula with formaldehyde caused the cores to harden, or freeze dry, more rapidly, so they didn't have to be baked.

Dad explained how everything in the core room was dusty, including dust on the framework ledges about a half-inch thick. The dust was generated by the sand mix formula which contained corn flour and oils. Also, workers continually brushed the cores with whisk brooms and filed chips off them. Then, the cores were dipped in a water solution to harden the surfaces. Finally, the cores were rotated in ovens to dry them.

Some ovens dried the cores and other ovens baked them. This process also stirred up a lot of dust. Dad said he believed the vertical ovens could have been insulated with asbestos. The dryers had large boards, 1½ to 2 inches thick, on which to set the cores. These boards could stand the heat because they were made of asbestos and another mineral.

Mr. Contrada asked, "Did you work around raw bags of asbestos?"

Dad answered, "I can't say that I did."

"Were there any warning signs posted that said you should wear a respirator for protection around asbestos?" Mr. Contrada wondered.

"There were no such signs. I don't remember respirators the first twenty years I worked there. They didn't come out and say much about them. After 1965, I sometimes wore a mask while painting. On real dirty jobs, I wore a respirator from the stock room, by my own choice. It had a rubberized thing around the nose and a string which went around the back of the head. The end where you could change the filters was cotton, about three by two inches in size and oval-shaped. The respirator would filter out dust, not chemicals. Hardly anyone wore a respirator when we first started," Dad concluded.

"Why were respirators available? Did anyone ever tell you?" inquired Mr. Contrada.

Dad responded, "No, they didn't."

"Were you aware that working around sand, you could get silicosis?" Mr. Contrada asked.

"Well, I never gave it much thought," Dad replied. "There were safety directors who would tell you to be careful around the trucks. You were told to keep your hands out of pinch points in the machinery. There was a state law about wearing ear plugs toward the last, but my hearing had already been damaged by then. Nothing was mentioned about the dangers of working with sand."

"Did you ever learn that asbestos could cause a disease or injury at the foundry?" Mr. Contrada wondered.

"I don't believe that I did. I never thought I was around it," Dad said.

Then, Mr. Contrada asked, "When did you first learn that asbestos causes serious disease?"

"I didn't know it caused cancer until I got it myself," Dad answered.

"You claim it happened on the job site. The defense is going to try to find every other place in your life where you could have been exposed. What about the service? Were you ever in the service?" asked Mr. Contrada.

Dad replied, "No...no."

Mr. Contrada concluded that we had potentially three claims.

One is a workman's compensation claim since the injury very likely occurred from exposure on the job. This claim would be filed against General Motors by another lawyer in the firm, Mr. Michael Dorf, who handles workman's comp cases.

The second claim would be against the manufacturers and processors of asbestos. These companies would be identified in an investigative search and by interviews with employees about what products were used at the foundry. Ninety percent of these claims are settled out of court, but there would be no guarantees and there is no typical settlement figure. Investigation could begin immediately. The only holdup would be locating the persons to interview.

The third claim would be against Johns-Manville's Trust. The Manville Corporation (formerly Johns-Manville), the largest asbestos company in the world, filed for bankruptcy in 1982. As part of the agreement and because of thousands of lawsuits brought against them by workers, the corporation set up a trust fund that could be paid to persons who were harmfully exposed to their products. An application called a proof of claim must be filed, and then, the claimee gets in a very long line behind others.

We also discussed with Mr. Contrada the names of persons who had worked at the foundry and were familiar with the work environment. Some were still employed, and others were retirees. Dad listed names of former workers who were deceased or currently had health problems. In fact, I had begun to notice the newspaper obituaries of former foundry employees whose deaths were due to cancer.

For a man who thought he had left the working conditions at Central Foundry behind him, my father had much to consider. Did he want to file a lawsuit because of his cancer? Should asbestos manufacturers be held accountable? Was using the criminal justice system an avenue he wanted to pursue?

Regarding annual chest X-rays at the foundry, Dad had signed a release form granting the foundry permission to send these X-rays to his doctors. Such a procedure to release medical records is regulated by state law. Dad had mailed the requests before his surgery in Seattle. Several years later, we have yet to receive a response or the X-rays from the foundry.

In addition, other retirees who knew they had worked around asbestos at the foundry asked my physician brother for referrals to a specialist. Lung and chest problems are more accurately found by a radiologist who is familiar with asbestos disease. The closest specialist lived in Toledo, an hour's drive from the foundry. Many workers wondered what their past chest X-rays had really revealed, since the foundry's medical personnel had never discussed the results with them.

I had my own beliefs about lawsuits to consider. It seemed we were living in a litigation society. Persons are constantly blaming others for their troubles. In my opinion, such blame had become excessive. Persons were actively looking for suspected problems, often in petty circumstances which could be settled by other means.

I was hesitant to share our problems in a public manner. Would others without similar problems understand what was happening? Would foundry employees become unnecessarily concerned about their own fate? I also wondered whether or not the employees would consent to be interviewed. These questions filled my thoughts and affected my mental state adversely.

On the other hand, my father was in an agonizing situation for which he had been given no warning. The disease and treatments were taking a progressive toll. We were not dealing with a cancer for which there was a light at the end of the tunnel. Instead, we had been told that Dad's condition would continually worsen. We did not know how soon the extensive tumors would debilitate him or how much pain the tumors would cause around sensitive nerves. Such thoughts further dampened my emotional state.

Mr. Contrada said that most victims were already deceased when their families filed lawsuits. We had the advantage of Dad's input and his desire to seek out the circumstances of his asbestos exposure. His own description of the work situation would be helpful. He would be able to take part in depositions.

I questioned why the producers of asbestos should still be doing business. If health dangers have been known for years, why had asbestos been used in thousands of buildings and products, especially in the fifties and sixties?

As a teacher, I knew that schools were required to have asbestos inspections and to finance the removal of a substance which had been deemed safe during their buildings' construction. School personnel may have scoffed at the supposed harm of asbestos as being another ploy of government regulation.

Well, I did know someone suffering from asbestos disease. And I wondered how much asbestos was in our daily environment that we have all been exposed to. Since there are no known safe levels, or limits, of exposure, I contemplated the number of future problems after the latency period. Persons with disease could have no idea where or when their past exposure happened. Is that what the asbestos companies had been counting on? Were government-imposed cutbacks occurring soon enough?

After much consideration, we decided to proceed with the lawsuits. Charles Contrada would begin the investigation as soon as Dad signed an agreement and gave authorization for release of medical and other data. The cause ahead of us became very important to my father.

Soon afterwards, we met with Michael Dorf about the workman's compensation case. Mr. Dorf explained that, like the suit against the manufacturers, it is necessary to prove there was asbestos in the foundry and that Dad's exposure took place there. Before the hearings, there would be an occupational safety investigation. The three levels of hearings included the district, the regional, and one by the Industrial Commission of Ohio. An unbiased doctor would examine Dad and his medical records. If a settlement is not reached, the suit could possibly go to trial. The suit would be against Central Foundry, the employer, because of exposure during the course of employment.

After filing for workman's compensation, a woman from the Industrial Commission of Ohio visited my parents. She asked questions about Dad's work situation and his physical incapacity because of disease.

In September of 1989, an asbestos investigator came to my parents' home to obtain basic information about Dad's work experience. Dad said he had worked in Department 710, or the core room, during his entire employment. When Dad was first hired, he was classified as a dryer man. He changed dryers on horizontal and vertical ovens. The dryers themselves were like a big slab, an inch or more thick and two by four feet in size, though some were smaller. The slabs contained asbestos to form a solid, heat-resistant board. Other dryers were just flat metal plates or odd shapes of aluminum.

The contour shape of the oven fit the cores. The outside of the ovens was a heavy gauge sheet metal, but the inside may have been insulated with asbestos. The ovens had cars swinging from tracks which were run by electric motor. Each car had a pulley in the middle and racks of shelves inside. The baking ovens were 400° Fahrenheit, while the drying ovens were 250° F. The foundry provided leather-faced gloves for protection and regular mitts for extremely hot things. Dad said he seldom used gloves.

In the core room, Dad was a dryer man, a core processor, an assembly line worker, a production inspector, and a relief man on similar work. On rare occasions, when the core room closed down,

Dad worked in the foundry, Dept. 112, or in Dept. 116, the finish department.

Dad explained that the foundry used to buy sand from Lake Michigan and haul it in. Big mixers mixed the sand formula so it had a consistency that would bake. The formula would then be fed from an overhead chute as it was poured to make cores. A pressurized machine came down to form the cores out of sand. Dad said the formula had to hold up in the flask (the frame used as a mold) about two minutes so that the hot metal could be poured.

After the cores were made, they were set in ovens and dryers of various shapes and sizes to support them. When the cores were cooled, the workers would shake them to remove sand. The sand could then be reused. Dad said he was around sand on a day to day basis, and the sand mixers were above his head.

The ovens had about sixty-four racks on them, each ten feet wide and two feet across. Rows of racks traveled over the tops of the ovens like a ferris wheel. Because the ovens were 30-35 feet high, they extended above the roof of the building.

To process the cores, Dad used a yellowish water-solution paint. He did this by dipping or spraying the cores with paint so that the hot metal would not penetrate the cores. Sometimes, he even mixed the paint by getting powders and clay out of barrels in the dip room. Then, he stirred in small amounts of water. He was unsure what the dry materials consisted of. The barrels also contained black and yellowish-green mud. Usually, workers classified as mixers would stir the paint mixture. Then, they would put it in tanks, haul it in big lift trucks, and pour it into dip vats.

Often, the ovens would get a build-up of water-solution paint from the processed cores. Because of this, Dad had to scrape the insides of the ovens. While the power was shut off, workers rode through the ovens to clean them.

In further interviews, Dad revealed that his employer had not designated face masks or respirators as asbestos protection.

The foundry had not been properly ventilated. No mention was made about disposable coveralls because of asbetsos exposure, and the gloves could have contained asbestos as well.

By the first of October, Dad and Mom were able to attend a dinner meeting of the retired United Auto Workers, Local 211, in which my father was an active member. The group meets monthly at the UAW Hall in Defiance, and 200-400 retirees and their spouses participate. Altogether, there are about 1,200 retirees. The law firm had contacted the union president and the foundry health inspector, and a program on asbestos in the workplace was planned. The program emphasized how to recognize symptoms of disease and why regular chest X-rays are needed to detect problems. The issue of asbestos concerned many retirees.

In attendance at the UAW meeting was our lawyer, Charles Contrada, and some of his investigative assistants. During one part of the meeting, my father was welcomed back from his recent surgery and treatments. At the program's conclusion, Mr. Contrada spoke about the kinds of physical problems my Dad was experiencing because of his asbestos exposure. Mr. Contrada asked if anyone present remembered specific asbestos products or label names in years past. He said such information would greatly help Dad and would be a source of information for the future.

After adjournment, union retirees lined up in unexpected numbers. Mr. Contrada and his assistants organized lines. They wrote as fast as they could, taking down workers' names, products, product labels, and companies which had supplied asbestos materials to the foundry. The retirees patiently waited to share their recollections from accumulated years of experience. They became a flowing source of information.

From that meeting and through further investigation, eighteen companies which had provided asbestos-related materials to the foundry were identified. Some companies were located in Ohio, some were in nearby states, several had changed their company name, and others were Canadian companies in the province of Quebec.

Construction of the Defiance foundry began in 1947, and the plant opened the summer of 1948. In the fifties, the employee ranks swelled to 5,000. When he retired in 1980, Dad thought there were about 4,000 workers and 300-400 salaried personnel. Because automation has taken over some tasks, there would now be about 2,500 employees.

One retiree, employed by the plant at its inception, said that 7,000 workers came and went during the first two to three years. The heavy turnover was due to the hard physical labor required.

The foundry site consists of three main sections, or plants. Plant 2 West was built beside the original factory in the mid-1960s. The third plant, Plant 2 East, was added about 1970. Renovations and construction took place every other year during peak years of the sixties and seventies. As a result, Dad said he constantly was exposed to dust from construction. Ventilation systems were only added to the plants recently.

Another retiree spoke about fellow workers who were now ill or who had already died of cancer. Many of them had worked in maintenance throughout the foundry. One example included a father and son who both contracted cancer. The man described how, as recently as the early 1980s, he handled asbestos by shoveling broken bricks containing asbestos into a hopper. A supervisor had given orders for his shift to do the job after the previous shift had refused. Afterwards, he said their clothes were burned.

Before an Open House or whenever a General Motors division manager or the president of the board was expected to visit the foundry, much painting and extensive cleaning took place. The dirty, dusty atmosphere of the foundry was transformed into an unrecognizably clean environment. One time, when Ralph Nader toured the foundry, a smoke-eater on one of the cupolas was not working properly. Because of this, the cupola was shut down during Nader's visit.

Another man, who had worked in the lab, said he wore an apron and leggings made of asbestos. The covering was intended to protect him while he worked with various chemicals. When workers were being trained on dealing with harmful chemicals, a question about the safety of the asbestos clothing was raised by a worker. No response was given about the harmful effects of wearing asbestos.

One lab worker said he was given a respirator to wear because of exposure to lead. The respirator was loose-fitting and caused an uncomfortable facial rash. The medical director regularly tested his blood for lead content. However, the worker was never given any results from his annual chest X-rays.

It is known that workers in American industries were heavily exposed to asbestos in some occupational environments before the government began to regulate asbestos in 1970. Because of the period between exposure and onset of disease, more workers will be affected in the near future. Some workers may have worked near contaminated areas while others may have worked directly with asbestos. Once asbestos particles enter the body, they are lodged there permanently. To detect potential problems, it is advisable to have an expert radiologist interpret chest X-rays. Even though there are regulations controlling dust levels in industry, there is no known safe level of asbestos exposure.

Chapter 19
What Is Mesothelioma?

Before this cancer occurred in my father, I had never known that there were several different diseases caused by exposure to asbestos. In particular, I had never heard of the cancer called mesothelioma. When the surgeon informed us of the diagnosis, we had trouble remembering the term and also difficulty pronouncing it correctly. It took two or three weeks before we could consistently say mesothelioma with a degree of confidence. Even then, the hospital staff would confuse us by mispronouncing it.

Not knowing much about mesothelioma, I looked it up in medical books. There was usually a definition of cause and a description of the location, followed by the statement that mesothelioma was a particularly fatal tumor with death occurring within a year. Thus, during my father's illness, I had trouble discussing the disease.

By definition, diffuse malignant mesothelioma is a fatal tumor arising from mesothelial cells, or cells in the lining of the pleura (chest), peritoneum (abdomen), or pericardium (heart), (Mossman et al., 1990, 295).

A single layer of flat cells, called the visceral membrane (about 1 mm thick) surrounds the organs. This layer of cells is connected to a second layer called the parietal membrane. Together, these two layers form the mesothelium which surrounds and protects the organs. The mesothelium produces a thin film of fluid which lubricates the movements of the lungs within the body (NCI Pub. 85-1847, 1985).

The time between initial occupational exposure to asbestos and the diagnosis of disease is rarely less than twenty years and averages forty years (Gilson, 1972, 122). Case studies have indicated that only a brief contact can cause cancer decades later (Agran, 1977, 31). In the disease, asbestos fibers have traveled through the walls of the lungs or stomach and have lodged in the chest and abdominal cavity.

Diagnosis of mesothelioma is especially difficult. First, the disease does not initially produce symptoms or cause noticeable problems. One may think that the shortness of breath has some other cause. Other signs of disease are loss of weight and a dull, aching chest pain with fluid in the chest. Pleural thickening may be apparent on chest X-rays (Peters and Peters, 1980, B7). As with my father, unusual dark spots may also be visible on X-ray.

Ivory-colored tumors, which gradually move across the chest lining like a thin spider web, scar the tissue and cause fibrosis. In earlier stages, this does not readily show up on X-ray. The tumor may look more like the metastases (spread) of another tumor, and not the primary tumor itself. The tumors encase the lungs in a rubbery mass of tissue. The tumor spreads along the interlobar fissures and invades adjacent organs including the heart, diaphragm, and liver. It is also common for the tumor to spread to the lymph nodes and lungs. Metastases outside the chest cavity are rare (Merchant, 1986, 313-314).

The cells of the cancer take on a wide variety of appearances under the microscope. The cells may range from epithelial to sarcomatoid to mixed forms. The tumor may be mistaken for an inflammation or for adenocarcinoma, a cancer of the gland. Usually, an open thoracotomy, rather than just a needle biopsy, is needed to obtain enough tissue for diagnosis and to determine the asbestos fiber count (Mossman and Gee, 1989, 1723).

Even in late stages of the disease, symptoms may resemble chronic bronchitis or broncho-pneumonia, partly because of fluid build-up from tumor growth. Or the victim may actually contract pneumonia as a result of lowered resistance.

It is thought that 90 percent of male mesothelioma deaths and 70 percent of the female deaths are due to mesothelioma of the pleura. The second largest number of tumors arise from the lining of the abdomen, and the fewest number of tumors begin in the lining of the heart (NCI Pub. 85-1847, 1985).

Mesothelioma was once considered a rare disease (Agran, 1977, 25). The first case associated with asbestos exposure was in 1946. In 1960, the connection between asbestos exposure and mesothelioma was firmly established. Since then, cases of the disease have been reported in all major industrial countries (Merchant, 1986, 313).

When compared to annual lung cancer deaths, which were 130,000 in 1984, there were only about 1,500 cases of mesothelioma per year in the United States, in the fifteen years prior to

1984. The mortality rate from mesothelioma for all women and for men under age sixty-five has remained constant. However, there has been a regular increase in death rates for men over sixty-five. The cancer has increased in geographic places where asbestos is manufactured and where shipyards are located (Mossman and Gee, 1989, 1723). After World War II, the growing use of asbestos increased the number of cases occurring now, following the thirty to forty year time span after exposure.

It is thought that mesothelioma is more common among workers who were exposed to the crocidolite fiber. Crocidolite fibers are considered less soluble in lung tissue. Because of their needle-like shape, they can penetrate deeper into the lungs. Over time, the fibers fragment and spread magnesium. On the other hand, the round chrysotile fibers occur in bundles which can be intercepted in airway passages more easily. Therefore, chrysotile fibers may be more soluble in the body (Mossman and Gee, 1989, 1722-23). However, mesothelioma has been confirmed in many countries with other asbestos fibers besides crocidolite (Merchant, 1986, 291-295).

There seems to be no connection between cigarette smoking and the occurrence of mesothelioma. Smoking does not increase the chances of getting the disease. Lack of smoking doesn't prevent the onset of disease (Mossman et al., 1990, 295). However, the same cannot be said about smoking and asbestos-caused cancers of the lung, in which smoking is a factor (Merchant, 1986, 298).

In the body, the carcinogen asbestos works in multiple stages, including initiation and promotion. The initiators interact with the DNA of the cells to produce changes. Promoters, which cause spreading of cells, encourage malignancy and new formations, or differentiations, in the cells. With both initiators and promoters, asbestos is considered a complete carcinogen (Mossman et al., 1990, 297).

As an initiator, there is scientific evidence that asbestos induces chromosomal mutations. In his laboratory work, Thomas Hesterberg concluded that mineral dust induces cell changes in chromosomal mutation. J.F. Lechner and others showed that asbestos fibers alter the growth properties of normal mesothelial cells in humans. At first, he found the cells were non-tumorous, but new variant cells appeared later that did produce tumors. The normal regulators of the tumor cells were suppressed. Simply stated, he found that the tumor regulators may be suppressed because of chromosome mutations caused by the presence of asbestos fibers (Barrett et al., 1989, 83-85).

Mesotheliomas have been found among the household members of asbestos workers. Studies have linked asbestos fibers as the cause of cancer in victims whose family members came home wearing clothing and shoes covered with dust. The worker deposited this dust around the house. Also, regular clothing could have been laundered with asbestos-contaminated clothes (Castle man, 1986, 414)

Cases of mesothelioma have also been found in persons who lived near a factory which used asbestos. Asbestos fibers can easily travel a mile or more in the air. Research done in London in 1965 by Muriel Newhouse and Hilda Thompson traced the history of eighty-three mesothelioma cases. Most could be traced to asbestos on the job. But eleven of the victims had no exposure at work or home. The common factor found was that they lived within a half mile of a factory where asbestos was used. This conclusion brought new light to how carcinogens can be transmitted (Boyle, 1979, 106-107). .

Mesotheliomas are rarely found in children. However, this idea may be changing. As in drug use, the effects of exposure for children can occur in a much shorter time period than for adults. Growing bodies of young persons have higher metabolic rates and, therefore, they may be more susceptible to invading carcinogens. Our lawyer told us about the father of a small girl who insulated his daughter's playhouse with asbestos in order to winterize it. The girl succumbed to mesothelioma by the age of five. Another factor for children is that they come in close contact with crushed rock on playgrounds and roads during play activity. These places may contain rock with asbestos fibers.

As in my father's case, the most commonly used method for treatment of mesothelioma is a combination of radiation and Adriamycin chemotherapy. Thoracentesis, or draining of excess pleural fluid, can also be helpful. Most patients survive less than a year after diagnosis. The goal with treatment is to prolong the survival rate and to make the patient more comfortable. No effective curative treatment is currently available.

During surgery, Dad had as much of the tumor removed as possible. The doctor also removed much of his cancer-ridden pleura. Because he no longer had the protective, lubricating layer of pleura, Dad experienced discomfort in his chest area when moving around or sitting too long in one position.

In retrospect on the years leading up to Dad's cancer, he experienced no noticeable breathing problems. He did, however, have a loud cough. When he caught a cold, it was usually severe and required a long time to dissipate.

Because of his otherwise excellent physical condition, we do not know how long it would have taken for the cancer symptoms to manifest themselves if the problem had not been discovered on X-ray. One doctor thought Dad could have had the cancer for six months to a year before diagnosis. Another doctor related that his mesothelioma patients lived only about two months after symptoms indicated the disease.

There are no specific tests to survey the occurrence of mesothelioma in the general population. Workers with known asbestos exposure should have periodic chest X-rays and lung function tests. Again, there is the difficulty of diagnosis, especially of not being able to detect the disease until it has spread. Preventative measures against exposure are still the best choice in avoiding the disease.

Chapter 20
Diminishing Respiratory Capacity

There are other serious diseases besides mesothelioma which are caused by asbestos exposure. These diseases include asbestosis, lung cancer, and cancers in other organs such as the esophagus, larynx, stomach, colon, and rectum. The diseases are progressive, irreversible, and incurable. Diagnosis of the diseases is difficult because the symptoms are nonspecific and ambiguous. Asbestos can also cause benign changes in the pleura and asbestos corns.

Asbestosis, nicknamed "white lung," is caused by asbestos fibers which have become embedded in the lungs. The disease was first diagnosed officially as "pulmonary asbestosis" in an English textile worker in 1924. In asbestosis, the irritating asbestos fibers cause scarring, or pleural, alveolar, and interstitual fibrosis, which reduce the elasticity of the lungs and limit the ability of the lungs to expand and contract. Along with fibrosis, excess deposits of collagen cause progressive lung stiffening and reduced gas exchanges. Unusual rales in the chest become audible. Scar tissue replaces healthy tissue to the extent that fibrous tissue blocks the lungs, and the victim becomes disabled and eventually suffocates (Mossman et al., 1990, 295).

Asbestosis is not a pleural cancer, as is mesothelioma, but it is a chronic lung disease with a gradual fibrosis of the lung tissues. Another difference is that the symptoms of asbestosis become apparent much earlier, perhaps with as little as ten years of exposure, and they last over a period of years. Symptoms gradually worsen, even without further asbestos exposure. So asbestosis may cause years of suffering and impaired breathing.

According to the American Cancer Society, symptoms of asbestosis include dyspnea (shortness of breath), a change in cough patterns, pain and tightness in the chest, difficulty in swallowing, weight loss, and ultimately, respiratory failure. Victims are more susceptible to colds, flu, and infections. The late stages can also produce swollen fingers and toes.

In a chest X-ray, asbestosis resembles fibrosis of the narrow places between tissues and reveals basal, irregular shadows. Shadows are more common among asbestos workers who smoke. The size and number of lesions help classify the disease as asbestosis.

Asbestosis was a predominant occupational disease from 1930-1955. At first, scientists and doctors thought the disease was a limited problem and could be controlled by reducing dust levels in factories. However, it has been prominent among asbestos workers who mine asbestos, manufacture asbestos products, or work in the building industry. Currently, there are thought to be 65,000 diagnosable cases in the United States (Sun, 1986, 543). Newly diagnosed cases are relatively mild when compared to cases 40-50 years ago (Mossman and Gee, 1989, 1726).

Asbestosis is not considered a threat outside the work environment. Today, the incidence is decreasing because of current dust level standards. Lung function tests are needed for detection and for assessment of diminished breathing capacity due to lung impairment.

Tumors causing asbestos lung cancer can arise from epithelial cells in the trachea, the bronchi, or the air sacs in the lungs. The symptoms are similar to asbestosis and may include coughing up blood, a rapid weight loss, chest pain, and fever from attacks of pneumonia and bronchitis. The tumors are often found on the lower lobes of the lungs. Receiving an early diagnosis and having surgery increase the survival time (Peters and Peters, 1980, B8).

The average latency period for lung cancer is somewhat less than for mesothelioma. Lung cancer can appear 15-25 years after asbestos exposure. Various factors which produce lung cancer are the type and composition of the fiber, the level of exposure, a worker's smoking habits, and other chemicals present in the work place. Lung cancers are highest in those exposed to amphibole fibers and lowest in chrysotile fiber workers (Mossman and Gee, 1989, 1722-1724).

There is some thought that the presence of asbestosis can cause lung cancer. Scar tissues have been known to occur at sites of inflammatory fibrosis. In many cases, both diseases have been found together. Whether asbestosis is a precursor of lung cancer victims or victims with asbestosis live long enough to contract both diseases is not fully known.

Smoking cigarettes increases the risk of developing lung cancer in persons exposed to asbestos. There is a much greater risk than by just smoking cigarettes alone. In 1982, the American Cancer Society stated that smokers may be up to ninety times more likely to develop lung cancer than unexposed non-smokers. When comparing asbestos workers who smoke and those workers who do not, smokers have a fifty times greater chance of developing lung cancer (Skinner et al., 1988, 138). Since asbestos impairs the lung's ability to clear fibers, smoking may magnify the extent of fibrosis. A problem in correlating smoking with asbestos workers is that many of the workers are also heavy smokers or are around heavy secondary smoke (Mossman and Gee, 1989, 1724).

Cancers of the gastrointestinal tract and the larynx have also been reported in large numbers among asbestos workers. This would make sense because asbestos fibers can be swallowed and would end up in the digestive system. Also, pipes lined with asbestos transport much of the nation's water supply.

Only a few asbestos diseases are affected by smoking cigarettes. Besides lung cancer, smoking along with asbestos exposure affects cancers of the esophagus, larynx, cheek cavity, and pharnyx. As stated previously, smoking does not affect mesothelioma. Smoking is also unrelated to cancers of the stomach, colon, rectum and kidney (Rothstein, 1984, 33).

There are four types of benign pleural disorders caused by asbestos. These include benign pleural effusions (fluid in the pleura), pleural plaques, pleural fibrosis, and atelectasis, or collapsed lung tissue. Scientists are unsure how asbestos fibers are carried to the pleura (Mossman et al., 1990, 295).

Benign pleural effusions occur in few workers twenty years after first exposure. About a third of these workers have pleural pain and shortness of breath. Most effusions go away, but some have been known to recur. Pleural thickening may also accompany the effusions.

Pleural plaques, or localized fibrous thickenings, are the most common benign problem to arise in the pleura. The plaques appear as glassy, fibrous, nodular lesions. Usually, they are located in the parietal layer, but can also occur in the linings of the diaphragm and the heart. Because of their location, the lesions do not commonly cause loss of lung function. Calcification of the lesions takes place over time, but doesn't indicate the lesions are growing bigger. On X-ray, pleural plaques can appear to be tumors or asbestosis lesions.

There is no evidence that benign pleural problems caused by asbestos exposure will eventually cause asbestosis or cancer

(Mossman and Gee, 1989, 1726-1727).

Asbestos can cause chronic skin irritations called asbestos corns. Needle-like asbestos fibers penetrate the skin, especially the hands. Skin cancer is not induced, however, and the asbestos corn can be excised (Peters and Peters, 1980, B10).

Through research, it was discovered that there might be a dosage-dependent factor with asbestos disease. Heavier doses in a short time may bring on disease sooner. Lighter exposure over a long period of time may also cause disease. However, like other carcinogens, asbestos can be dangerous at very low levels (Boyle, 1979, 106).

There is disagreement about whether or not the size of the asbestos fiber influences disease. Long and thin fibers may be more carcinogenic than short, thick ones. Because some fibers are less durable and dissolve more easily in the body, such fibers might cause fewer problems. The chemical makeup of the fiber may also be a factor in causing disease (Mossman et al., 1989, 296).

Some scientists think the short fibers from .5 to 5 microns penetrate the alveoli and bronchioles more easily. Small fibers could penetrate all the way to the pleura while medium length fibers would end up in the higher respiratory passages. As the immune system attacks the ingested fibers, the fibers eventually become encapsulated asbestos bodies, or fibrous tissue, in the air sacs of the lungs.

At the present time, diseases caused by asbestos cannot be effectively treated. Avoiding exposure to any amount of the fibers or dust is the best solution. Those who work with asbestos need specially fitted respirators and other precautions. Persons who continue to smoke are inviting trouble. Persons who already have scarred lung tissue should have regular vaccines to prevent flu and pneumonia.

Chapter 21
Using the White, Magic Mineral

Asbestos is the name for a naturally occurring family of minerals which are mined from metamorphic rocks and composed of tiny fibers. Asbestos began its formation millions of years ago from rocks which broke through the earth's crust. These breaking points filled with mineral-rich water which made veins in the rocks. After years of pressure and heat, the veins crystallized into masses of mineral fibers.

The fibers, or threads, can easily break, stick to clothing, and float in the air. If the fibers become airborne, they can be inhaled or swallowed, and thus lodged in the lungs or abdomen indefinitely. The word asbestos is derived from Greek and means "inextinguishable." The fibers of this silicate mineral are strong and immune to heat, yet delicate and flexible to use.

The unique qualities of asbestos were noted by early Romans who used the fibers in woven cloth and in lamp-wicks. The indestructible characteristics of asbestos were rediscovered during the Industrial Revolution of the late nineteenth century in Europe and America.

The family of asbestos fibers can be divided into two main classes: serpentine fibers and amphibole fibers. The most common serpentine fiber is chrysotile which is used in 90-95 percent of the world's asbestos production. Chrysotile fibers are curly and resemble tubular scrolls. They are so fine and strong that a pound of fiber can yield 30,000 feet of thread. Chrysotile contains mainly silica, magnesium, and water.

The amphibole fibers are more diverse and are used less in industry. These fibers, characterized by their needle shape, are composed of magnesium, calcium, sodium, and iron. Examples of them include crocidolite (blue asbestos), amosite (an acronym for Asbestos Mines of South Africa), actinolite, tremolite, and anthophyllite. Various types of asbestos fibers differ in their composi-

105

tion and durability. Sophisticated technology such as electron microscopy is required to identify specific types of asbestos fibers.

Asbestos has been widely used in industry because of its resistance to heat and acid, its durability, and its low cost. Before the turn of the century, it was popularly used as a heat insulator for boilers, ovens, and steam pipes. Asbestos fibers were also used in the textile industry, both in England and the United States. Since the early 1900s, the use of asbestos has increased many times over. However, since that time, it has been known that the inhalation of asbestos fibers caused disabling diseases of the lungs (Brodeur, 1985, 11).

The use of asbestos in the space industry and in defense escalated during World War II. In the postwar building boom, asbestos became a standard element in floors, ceilings, pipes, and furnaces. The versatile nature of asbestos, as a fire-retardant, brought about the nickname, "the white, magic mineral."

Total world production each year is nearly five million tons. Canada, the largest producer of asbestos, exports millions of dollars worth per year, much of it to Third World countries where health standards are not as strict. Canadian exports to the United States have dropped drastically since the seventies. In recent years, the former Soviet Union has expanded its Siberian asbestos mining, and competes with Canada as the leader in the amount of production.

Mines near the town of Asbestos in Quebec, Canada, provide most of the world's supply of chrysotile. This huge deposit, which is seventy miles long and six miles wide, was discovered in 1860 and has been mined since 1878. Other large deposits of asbestos ore are located in South Africa and the former Soviet Union. In fact, deposits in the Ural Mountains prompted the first asbestos manufacturing factory in the eighteenth century. The United States now has very few profitable sources, although asbestos has been mined in California, Arizona, and Vermont.

The most common method of obtaining asbestos is open-pit mining, usually for chrysotile. It can also be mined in tunnels by blasting. After the fibers are separated from the ore by various processes, they are drawn through screens and graded according to length. The length and composition of the fiber determine what products can be made from them.

Use of asbestos grew so rapidly that it was used in over three thousand domestic and industrial products during its peak. Its biggest use was in construction as a fireproofing material and insulator. It was also used in shingles, roofing, ceiling panels, floor tiles, electrical wires, textured paints, and wallboards (Boyle, 1979, 106).

An estimate by the Environmental Protection Agency is that over 730,000 public and private buildings contain asbestos materials. That figure does not include the thousands of schools built from 1940-73. In addition, asbestos is found in millions of homes such as in ducts for heating and cooling systems. As structures with asbestos age, the asbestos can crumble into microscopic fibers and cause future health problems. Before EPA warnings in 1973, over thirty million tons of asbestos had been used in building. Workers were exposed initially, and are re-exposed every time there is maintenance or repair work done. Whole neighborhoods are exposed when buildings are torn down. (Castleman, 1986, 615-616).

Other uses of asbestos involved the automotive industry. They made products such as drum brake linings, clutch pads, gaskets, and transmission components.

Cement pipes containing asbestos were used in pipes for sewers, drainage, irrigation, and water mains. Additional products which made use of the heat resistant capability of asbestos were pot holders, ironing board covers, hair dryers, artificial fireplace logs, theater curtains, conveyor belts, and fireproof apparel.

During World War II, about four and a half million shipyard workers inhaled large quantities of asbestos fibers. Dad's surgeon in Seattle had referred to cases of disease there. The workers had applied insulation to pipes and surfaces in the holds of ships and to engine hulls and decks. Asbestos was also used on pipes and boilers in other war-related industries. Because of the latent period between exposure and occurrence of disease, many shipyard workers began suffering problems in the sixties and seventies.

Asbestos expert, Dr. Irving Selikoff, estimated that about twenty-five million Americans have been exposed to significant amounts of asbestos on the job. This exposure took place from World War II to about 1980. Dr. Selikoff thinks there will be 270,000 deaths from asbestos-related cancers within the next twenty years (Brodeur, 1985, 258). Another source estimates that a death will occur every sixty minutes (WBGH TV, 1984). Others consider this a conservative guess, considering the numbers in the general population who have also experienced exposure.

Asbestos is the biggest industrial problem known in the field of occupational health. By comparison, other industrial problems have killed hundreds, while asbestos has killed thousands. It not only affects workers who made the products, but scores of persons who later used the products. Even brief contact has been known to cause cancer twenty to forty years later. According to the National Institute for Occupational Safety and Health, or NIOSH, there is no scientifically known safe level of exposure.

How long have health hazards from asbestos exposure been observed? According to records, a factory inspector in England warned workers about exposure in a health report issued in 1898. In 1900, a London physician autopsied a worker in an asbestos textile factory. Fibers were found in his lung tissues, and his death was attributed to severe pulmonary fibrosis. The deceased man was a member of a team who all died at the average age of thirty.

The first recorded death due to asbestosis, a respiratory illness which gradually decreases the victim's ability to breathe, was in 1924. Dr. W. E. Cooke, who wrote about the woman in the *British Medical Journal*, was the doctor who named the disease, "pulmonary asbestosis." His article was titled, "Fibrosis of the Lungs Due to Inhalation of Asbestos Dust." The autopsy revealed fibrous tissue connecting the lungs and the pleural membrane. The woman, who died at age thirty-three, had worked in a textile mill for twenty years.

Even in the United States, doctors had noticed lung scarring on the lungs of asbestos workers as early as 1917. In 1918, an insurance company refused to insure a client because they claimed asbestos might cause physical harm. And in 1927, the first workman's compensation claim was filed in Massachusetts by a man suffering from asbestosis.

In England, an historic report was produced in 1930 after an investigation of conditions in the asbestos industry. The government-sponsored survey was headed by Dr. E.R.A. Merewether, Medical Inspector of Factories. Major medical journals published the results.

Merewether had examined 363 asbestos workers actively employed in the asbestos textile industry. From this group, he discovered that over one-fourth, or ninety-five, definitely had asbestosis, while twenty-one others showed beginning signs of the disease. Incidence of disease increased proportionally when considering the number of years employment. None of the workers employed under five years had a diagnosable problem, but four out of five workers with twenty or more years of experience did have asbestosis.

Dr. Merewether noticed that chest X-rays of diseased workers had a diffuse, hazy appearance. His descriptions of lung fibrosis could have been taken from my father's own medical records. If this information was medically known and substantiated in 1930, why had the manufacturers of asbestos proceeded to escalate their sales of the white, magic mineral?

Following his investigation, Merewether made suggestions to the textile industry for reducing dust exposures and educating the workers. Thus, in 1931, England became the first country to establish health laws regulating asbestos exposure. Merewether concluded that being removed from the work environment after exposure did not keep the disease from causing further deteriorating health, since the fibers were already trapped in the lungs.

In 1929, the asbestos industry asked the Metropolitan Life Insurance Company to study whether or not asbestos dust was an occupational problem, and if it was, what measures could be taken to control the problem. In the findings on 126 persons randomly selected from asbestos plants, 53 percent of the X-rays showed asbestosis, and another 31 percent had signs of the disease. Only the remaining 16 percent had no sign of asbestosis.

Metropolitan Life, influenced by attorneys from Johns-Manville Corporation, ignored these statistics and made no recommendation that the industry be regulated in the United States. The results of the study were not published for four years, and the published version had been weakened in its message. Metropolitan Life did make suggestions that the problem of dust control be faced, that employees be given bi-annual chest X-rays, and that the industry could study the effect of asbestos on the body.

In 1938, Nordmann published a paper in Germany called "The Occupational Cancer of Asbestos Workers." Nordmann was the first to conclude that lung cancer affected asbestos workers. He projected the time period between exposure and resulting death as fifteen to twenty years. In these lung cancers, Nordmann found that tumors developed in the lower lobes of the lungs, whereas other known lung cancers generally began in the upper lobes. He discovered that there could be more than one primary site of malignancy in one person's lungs.

During this time, the United States was in the midst of the Depression, and people were just glad to find a job. They weren't worried about the problems of occupational health. Public concern and scientific data about asbestos workers was displaced by struggles of the Depression and the ensuing involvement of the United States in World War II.

In Germany in 1943, Dr. H.W. Wedler reported that there were pleural and lung tumors being found along with asbestosis. In world-wide writings, about 15 percent of asbestos-related autopsies also revealed lung and pleural tumors. At the time, this incidence surpassed lung cancer statistics for the general population which were only 2 to 6 percent.

Dr. Anthony Lanza, Assistant Medical Director for Metropolitan Life, asserted that all the business about chemicals causing cancer would soon be over. He said that the publication of studies linking asbestos to cancer would frighten people and cause asbestos companies unfair publicity. The studies were published anyway. But since researchers had to contend with pressure from asbestos companies, research was being curtailed at the expense of furthering knowledge.

By 1954, asbestos victims were living longer as a result of more regulations over dust levels. In twenty years, the average age of victims had increased from age forty to age fifty-five. However, it was found that persons with asbestosis were now living long enough to also have pulmonary cancer. In one series of autopsies, one-fourth of the cases had cancer of the lung as well as asbestosis.

At a conference on environmental carcinogens, sponsored by the National Cancer Institute, a panel of experts concluded that some studies had suggested a relationship between asbestos and lung cancer, but no reliance could be placed on them, and there had been too few laboratory investigations from which to draw conclusions. One of the "expert" members of the panel was the medical director of the Johns-Manville Corporation.

Many cases of cancer related to asbestos were reported in the late 1950s. By 1955, a number of medical journals had documented cases of mesothelioma of the pleura occurring in the United States, Canada, and Europe. Not until 1960, when South Africa reported thirty-three cases of mesothelioma in workers from crocidolite mines, was asbestos considered the cause of mesothelioma. Other mesothelioma victims were found among construction and shipyard workers.

Around 1960, the connection between asbestos and cancer was definitely established by research at Mount Sinai School of Medicine. Researchers proved that asbestos caused mesothelioma, the rare and fatal cancer of the lining of the lungs or abdomen (Winter, 1979, 34).

During the previous forty years, the asbestos industry sponsored several studies which established a relationship between asbestos fibers and asbestosis and cancer. Often, however, the results were not shown to the public or were published in altered form. Industrial efforts to withhold knowledge took place while the use of asbestos greatly increased. Lack of information delayed government efforts to regulate dust levels and, in turn, increased the number of persons exposed to higher levels.

Dr. Wilhelm C. Hueper said that the hesitance of the Public Health Service to respond to occupational cancer prevention was due to political influence. Interference by asbestos manufacturers provided an avenue for personal greed and corruption. Management influenced physicians to control costs for illness and injury at work. Physicians created the pretense of maintaining the health of workers.

Little information about regulating employees' exposure to asbestos was published before 1970. However, the demand for industrial physicians had grown rapidly. Until the passage of the Occupational Safety and Health Act (OSHA) in 1970, United States government inspectors could not enter general industrial work places. Before then, the Public Health Service depended on industry to carry out its own health studies. According to Dr. Hueper, the Public Health Service restricted research on occupational cancer in 1951 because of pressure from industry.

In 1972, the Occupational Safety and Health Act adopted the U.S. standards for all industries. The asbestos emission standards are "two fibers per cubic centimeter." The Environmental Protection Agency's standard is "no visible emission."

In 1978, the U.S. Secretary of Health, Education, and Welfare, Joseph Califano, Jr., stated that asbestos was a potent carcinogen and a producer of lung diseases. He ordered the Surgeon General of the United States to advise all physicians in the nation of the health risks of asbestos exposure. He also urged asbestos workers to stop smoking cigarettes (Brodeur, 1985, 140-141).

By 1980, OSHA had issued regulations for only twenty substances. OSHA acknowledged that its health standards were based on guidelines by industry rather than research of its own. In 1982, the American Cancer Society made the following resolution:

> There is a large body of accumulated scientific evidence that occupational exposure to asbestos fibers increases the risk of developing asbestosis, lung cancer, mesothelioma, and cancer of several other sites. Other exposures to asbestos may also be hazardous, such as those in environmental and household contact circumstances. The American Cancer Society urges that all human exposure to asbestos be minimized. The American Cancer Society is continuing to support research to determine the extent of such risk. People occupationally exposed to asbestos should be made aware of such hazards and appropriate control measures should be employed (American Cancer Society, 1982).

Asbestos is in the air we breathe and the water we drink. It has been documented in water supplies and food products, in drugs and in cosmetics. It is found in our homes and in public buildings. Asbestos becomes airborne when buildings are torn down. Fibers also become airborne when brake linings on cars wear out or when we drive on roads which have asbestos ore. Asbestos is in the products we use. It can be found in the lungs of the population in general, including children.

Certain occupations have involved more risk of exposure and need for regulation. Some of these include cement pipe makers, automobile mechanics, building construction and demolition workers, electricians, engineers, insulation workers, machinists, oil refinery workers, pipe and furnace fitters, plumbers, road builders, school maintenance personnel, and welders (Fletcher, 1988, 32).

People die every day from diseases caused by asbestos. Many of these persons were exposed unknowingly years ago. The fibers that caused their problems cannot be seen by the naked eye. Some deaths could have been avoided by limiting exposure or wearing protective apparel. Asbestos is truly a monumental concern of the twentieth century.

Chapter 22
Regulating a Carcinogen

Although hazards from asbestos exposure were recognized at the turn of the century, it wasn't until 1970 that asbestos was considered a major health concern in the United States. As a result of the Occupational Safety and Health Act of 1970, the government created agencies with the goal of promoting safe and healthy working conditions. All three agencies, including the Occupational Safety and Health Administration, the National Institute for Occupational Safety and Health, and the Environmental Protection Agency, have been involved in formulating regulations for asbestos.

The Occupational Safety and Health Administration, or OSHA, is an agency of the U.S. Department of Labor. Its chief task is to develop and enforce safety and health regulations on the job. The regulations deal with fire safety and protective clothing as well as maximum levels of exposure to toxic substances. OSHA sends inspectors to check industries for violations. Businesses argue that OSHA regulations are too costly, while labor leaders claim the standards lag behind needed changes.

The National Institute for Occupational Safety and Health, or NIOSH, is an agency of the U.S. Department of Health and Human Services. Its investigators study work conditions where there have been illnesses or accidents. After researching potentially dangerous situations, NIOSH recommends standards for work conditions. Because NIOSH reports its findings to OSHA, it has no enforcement authority. It does approve safety equipment such as respirators and provides training for job safety and health.

The Environmental Protection Agency, or EPA, was established in 1970 and is an independent agency of the government. The EPA establishes and enforces environmental protection standards, conducts research, provides grants, and recommends policies to the U.S. President.

According to Dr. David Fletcher in his 1988 article from *Medical Self-Care,* more than 200,000 deaths from lung cancer have been related to asbestos. In the 1990s, there is a strong likelihood of 150,000 asbestos deaths. Most deaths, so far, have been due to occupational exposure. About 1.5 million persons are currently exposed in the work place. In addition, there is disease in families of asbestos workers and in neighborhoods where factories and buildings contain asbestos.

Specialists in occupational health agree that nearly everyone has had some degree of consumer and environmental contact. Asbestos regulations for consumer products and for the environment have been minimal. The enormous use of asbestos, before government curtailment, expanded the risks of disease from a few thousand workers to millions of persons in the general population.

Even if all mining and use of asbestos stopped, there would still be air contamination because of the disintegration of already existing fibers. Examples of everyday exposures include maintenance workers who work in contaminated buildings, auto workers who repair brakes, and occupants who live in buildings where there are pipes lined with asbestos material. In 1963, a pathologist in South Africa discovered asbestos bodies occurring routinely in the lungs of urban dwellers (Castleman, 1986, 413).

The lung defenses cannot deal with the indestructible fibers, and no level of asbestos dust is so low that the lung fails to retain some fibers. Levels of dust which don't cause asbestosis can, however, cause cancer. And the amount needed to cause asbestosis is not as great as once thought. Persons can develop asbestosis from a brief, intense exposure or from a prolonged accumulation over years (Castleman, 1986, 406-408).

Consumption of asbestos in the United States reached a peak in the year 1973 at 795,000 metric tons. Since then, its use has fallen each year. United States use was 120,000 metric tons in 1986, the first time it had been that low since 1934. By 1989, asbestos use was down to 85,000 metric tons in the United States.

World consumption of asbestos has reached a plateau of 4.5 to 4.8 metric tons. Concerned industrial nations are using less, while developing countries are increasing their use. Knowledge about asbestos hazards varies from total ignorance to far-reaching alarm. Even though the United States has banned asbestos insulation, American companies continue to produce and market it in places such as Brazil and India. With the known dangers, it seems criminal to continue production without efforts to educate and protect foreign workers.

Through investigations and reports as early as the 1930s, major U.S. corporations, which mined and manufactured asbestos, became aware that breathing asbestos fibers could cause a fatal disease. Beginning in 1929, corporations conducted studies involving medical tests and air samplings. Johns-Manville executives told another asbestos firm in the 1940s that the financial loss of informing their workers about disease would be too great in terms of unrest and compensation claims.

Corporate efforts to withhold knowledge from workers indirectly kept the knowledge of asbestos hazards from the scientific community and the general public. This took place during a dramatic increase in asbestos use and, in turn, an increase in the number of endangered persons.

Johns-Manville Corporation's concern about the problem of asbestosis dates back to the twenties, when officials asked Dr. Anthony Lanza to do a health survey. Factual summaries of British medical reports can be found in a Johns-Manville communication from 1930. As early as 1929, lawsuits were filed against Johns-Manville, and an asbestosis lawsuit settlement was reached in 1933.

During the years 1930-1950, Vandiver Brown, corporate attorney for Johns-Manville, handled health hazards of asbestos. The activities of Brown are known through the Sumner Simpson Papers. They include making editorial suggestions for Dr. Lanza's research studies, discouraging the trade magazine *Asbestos* from printing stories on dust control or asbestosis, and representing asbestos companies who sponsored research at the Saranac Laboratory in New York. In the latter, Brown convinced the researcher to omit all mention of cancer in his reports.

As a member of asbestos organizations, Johns-Manville continually attended meetings and received publications about asbestos disease. In 1954, Hugh M. Jackson, the corporate safety manager, wrote to an Illinois plant that compliance with the threshold limit values for employee exposure did not assure protection for all workers. In 1950, the Saranac Lab reviewed cases of asbestosis and lung cancer for Johns-Manville.

Raybestos-Manhattan, Inc., was another leading manufacturer of asbestos products. Renamed Raymark in 1982, the company has produced friction products since the twenties. The company has admitted paying compensation to employees for disability from asbestosis since the thirties.

Raybestos-Manhattan brought to light what have become the best known discovery documents in asbestos litigation. The revealing corporate documents, known as the Sumner Simpson Papers, involve the correspondence and file reports of Sumner Simpson, president of the company in the thirties and forties. He exchanged letters with attorney Vandiver Brown of Johns-Manville. The letters show a pattern of denial which included knowledge of disease and suppression of evidence.

The Sumner Simpson Papers show, in writing, that the two companies held editorial say over publication of the first asbestos study by the industry in 1935. The papers display a conscious effort to keep information from employees and the public for fear of lawsuits. Omitted material from a 1935 study included, "It is possible for uncomplicated asbestosis to result fatally."

In the Sumner Simpson Papers, there are thousands of pages documenting the non-publication of asbestosis articles. The companies okayed animal studies with the agreement that the results would be considered industry property. The papers provide records of dust counts for various processes, including where values were over the limits. The results reveal that Simpson was aware in the thirties of Public Health Service studies on asbestosis. More recent documentation shows that the company admitted not knowing what a safe level of exposure was (Castleman, 1986, 464-472).

Members of the occupational medical profession have also been suspect. There have been attempts to prevent enforcement of the Occupational Safety and Health Standards. The physicians were also in complicity for refusing to publish medical information which might subject their employer to lawsuits. Perhaps, they have also been involved, along with industry, in blaming nonoccupational sources for occupational disease (Rothstein, 1984, 4).

There is currently a need for specialties with training in recognizing illnesses caused by occupational exposure. One solution would be to not subject physicians to managerial judgments or conflicts of interest. Workers themselves need to be educated. There is a need to improve workplace conditions with more detailed medical surveillance, and not just tests conducted to avoid civil liability (Rothstein, 1984, 202-204).

OSHA's asbestos standard requires an annual medical examination for each employee exposed to airborne concentrations of asbestos fibers. The examination must include a chest X-ray, a medical history for symptoms of respiratory disease, and a pulmonary function test. This exam is also required to be given either thirty days before or after the end of employment.

Many physicians are not able to diagnose asbestos disease. A chest X-ray should be examined by a B-reader, a radiologist who has been certified by the International Labor Organization for identifying occupationally related diseases. The X-rays should be checked for evidence of fibrosis, tumors, pleural plaques, and benign asbestos growths. A pulmonary function test should be done.

If a problem is suspected, further examination could include tests to measure gas exchanges, tests to measure lung function during exercise, and a biopsy of the lung, if needed. The tests should be provided annually to any workers exposed to levels of .1 fiber per cubic centimeter or higher (Fletcher, 1988, 32).

Currently, there are thousands of legal cases pending against manufacturers of asbestos. Persons with disease may file product liability actions which allege negligence, implied warranties, and misrepresentation. These third party lawsuits are filed against manufacturers, distributors, installers, and contractors of asbestos products.

Common allegations against the defendants are that they failed to provide adequate warnings, and they failed to inform workers to wear protective equipment and avoid contaminated air. Another allegation is that testing was not done to determine the product's risks. And, after ascertaining that the product could cause disease, the defendants failed to remove the product from the marketplace. Also, various defendants ignored or actively hid medical and scientific data, distorted medical examinations, refused to publish adverse test results, gave out misleading scientific studies, and misrepresented the nature and extent of the danger (Peters and Peters, 1980, D 1-D 4).

Because of the latency period of the disease, the plaintiff has several problems when filing a lawsuit. While in a state of progressive illness, the disease victim is forced to delve into his work background. He has the burden of identifying products and company names which were common 30-40 years previously. Because the products were not labeled as harmful, the worker may not have a clear idea about what they contained. If he wasn't in charge of the orders, he may not be knowledgeable about the companies involved. Purchase records may have been discarded or destroyed. Former fellow workers may be difficult to contact. The victim's industry may be uncooperative and may not want publicity about such claims to influence other employees.

Arguments which have been used by the asbestos companies in their defense are that low levels of exposure are not harmful, that cigarette smoking was a causative factor, that the ill person was exposed in some other setting such as the military, or that there was not a long enough exposure period. Companies have claimed that they had no knowledge of the disease hazard before 1964, even though documents and medical literature show otherwise. The manufacturers also attempt to claim that it was the contractor's duty to warn consumers if the product being installed was dangerous.

The Manville Corporation (formerly Johns-Manville), the world's largest asbestos mining and manufacturing firm, filed for bankruptcy on August 26, 1982. At that time, there were 16,500 asbestos-related lawsuits and an estimated 32,000 anticipated over the next twenty years. In 1982, Manville had $2 billion in annual sales and $1 billion in assets (Rothstein, 1984, 187). After filing under Chapter 11, Manville reported a profit of $43.6 million for the first half of 1983. In addition, by filing bankruptcy, Manville gained a half billion dollar subsidy from U.S. tax payers.

Manville has been affected by its escape to bankruptcy court. Manville had to cut prices in order to get business. Litigation still dominates the attention of top management. But filing bankruptcy provided Manville some time and restored profits.

In 1985, Manville established a Personal Injury Settlement Trust. Persons with health claims can sue the trust if unable to reach agreement. The trust was funded with $200 million in cash and $615 million in insurance settlement proceeds. It was also funded with a $1.65 billion non-interest bearing bond and 50 to 80 percent of Manville stock. Beginning the fifth year, Manville planned to contribute 20 percent of their own profits. Only a small amount in the trust was allotted for punitive damages and property claims. Manville was able to deduct the entire cost of the trust as a business expense.

In 1986, Manville unsuccessfully sued the United States government in an effort to force the government to share the burden of paying asbestos claims. Manville said that the government was a co-conspirator in limiting information about health dangers of asbestos during shipbuilding in World War II. Also, the asbestos industry attempted to sue the tobacco companies for joint liability in asbestos disease cases.

New claims continue to be filed against the trust. It was estimated that the trust had the potential of paying a top limit of 100,000 claims. During the first half of 1987, Manville stock dropped in value to two to three dollars a share.

In the fall of 1989, it was announced that the Manville Personal Injury Settlement Trust was in danger, by 1990, of running out of funds to pay asbestos victims. Selling the remaining 20 percent of its stock would cover the gap. By September of 1989, the trust fund had settled 15,485 claims and had 66,000 claims still pending. By 1991, the trust got $75 million annually from its bonds, and by 1992, the trust received up to 20 percent of the Manville profits (Atchison, 1989, 36).

Since 1977, asbestos company defendants in litigation have supported bills introduced in the U.S. Congress. These proposed bills would replace court-filed asbestos cases with a federally administered program. The asbestos companies and the government would fund the program together. Presumably, the motivation for such legislation proposals is to limit industry costs (Castleman, 1986, 626).

Legislation in England preceded that in the United States by fifty years. Beginning in 1898, hazards of asbestos were reported annually by the Chief Inspector of Factories. The first asbestos standards were published in 1931. These standards specified the use of breathing equipment, proper ventilation, protective clothing, and also prohibited employment of children. In 1969, British asbestos regulations detailed further requirements (Peters and Peters, 1980, D 28-D 29). A standard of 2 fibers per cubic centimeter for the chrysotile fibers was used in the seventies. A standard of 1 fiber/cc was adopted in 1983, and .5 f/cc in 1984 (Castleman, 1986, 584).

In earlier decades, there was no requirement for manufacturers in the United States to moniter employee asbestos exposure, and little data was published in the years 1930-70. The 5 MPPCF (millions particles per cubic foot) threshold limit value, issued by the Public Health Service in 1938, had been loosely followed. But, few state agencies had the authority to enforce those standards.

In 1970, the Occupational Safety and Health Administration set the first exposure limit for asbestos in the United States workplace at 12 fibers per cubic centimeter of air. This was to be reduced to 2 fibers/cc by July 1, 1976, with a ceiling limit of 10 fibers. However, in 1975, OSHA proposed lowering the exposure limit to .5 f/cc for an eight hour time-weighted day, with 5 f/cc for a ceiling limit (Castleman, 1986, 282-283).

When further studies showed such a level as unsafe, NIOSH recommended lowering the limit to .1 f/cc. After years of legal battles and petitions, OSHA issued a new exposure level of .2 f/cc and mandated medical surveillance programs for exposures over .1 f/cc (Fletcher, 1988, 32).

OSHA standards cover all asbestos-exposed workers. In the standards, a company is required to monitor the level of airborne asbestos and to document changing levels. Workers must wear properly-fitted respirators and protective clothing. There must be rooms where workers can remove contaminated clothing. Employers are required to provide annual physicals and to keep medical and exposure records for thirty years. Warning signs are to be posted in exposed areas and warning labels affixed to materials.

OSHA rulemaking is very complicated, and standards have been issued for only 24 substances since 1970. OSHA has issued a limited standard which requires putting identifying labels on chemicals in the workplace. OSHA regulations give present and past employees access to their medical records, exposure records, and company studies regarding employee work conditions. An OSHA advisory committee has considered the recommendation of a separate asbestos standard for the construction industry (Castleman, 1986, 583-584).

Other organizations have also dealt with asbestos regulations and studies. The Department of Labor supported research into projected mortality rates and economic effects of asbestos disease. Various navy documents discuss the hazards of asbestos in shipyards. The U.S. Department of the Interior has issued reports on substitutes for asbestos. The U.S. Consumer Product Safety Commission banned asbestos in some consumer products and summarized current information in other products. State laws on workman's compensation have provided a record of occupational diseases, causative agents, and hazardous industries.

Labels on asbestos products were a long time in coming. Some manufacturers of insulation products put caution labels on their products in 1964. In 1969, the first warning labels were applied to sacks of asbestos fibers. Warnings on asbestos cement and brake linings did not occur until the seventies.

OSHA requires that caution signs be posted at all approaches to areas with excessive concentrations of airborne asbestos fibers. OSHA specifies minimum letter sizes and has provided signs since 1979. The warning mentions asbestos as a dust void. It warns against staying in the area unless work requires it and wearing protective clothing. It does not specify disease, but states that "asbestos dust may be hazardous to your health."

OSHA requires caution labels on all products or containers with asbestos fibers, including raw material and debris. The label does not mention protective clothing, respirators, dust level control, care in handling, or what diseases may result from exposure. It has been suggested that using universal symbols instead of words would be more meaningful.

Removal of asbestos is one of the fastest growing businesses in America. The cost for removal is millions of dollars. Taxpayers are footing the bill for public buildings including removal from schools. Persons in commercial and residential buildings have to meet certain guidelines. An estimated 750 million tons of asbestos can be found in ceilings, walls, and attics of the nation's public buildings, especially in states with buildings which are insulated against cold weather (Sheler, 1987, 33). The real estate value of such buildings has dropped considerably.

Since approval of the Asbestos Hazard Emergency Response Act in 1986, Congress has authorized funds to help local governments inspect for asbestos, and encapsulate or remove it. Under this law, schools had until October of 1988 to inspect buildings and make plans for removal. Inspections had to be done by certified asbestos inspectors. Fifteen million school children and 1.4 million school workers have potentially been exposed (Sheler, 1987, 33). The estimated cost for removal per school building was about $90,000. Targeted were schools built from 1940-73 (Fletcher, 1988, 32).

As of November, 1989, thirty states had launched action against present and former asbestos manufacturers to recover cleanup costs for thousands of public buildings. Schools had to remove asbestos by July of 1989. When razing a structure, guidelines had to be followed. Eventually, all buildings with asbestos will need renovation, even though the asbestos doesn't pose an immediate problem (Bremner, 1989, 36-38).

The demand for asbestos removal service exceeds the new industry's ability to safely provide it. With $200 million in profits in 1983, the removal service's revenues for 1988 surpassed $2.7 billion. Poorly trained and equipped workers, however, can send additional asbestos particles into the air. Forty states have created training and certification programs for asbestos removal. The EPA is thinking about extending the 1986 Asbestos Hazard Emergency Response Act to include commercial and other public buildings (Whitaker, 1989, 53).

One study attacked the nation's asbestos policy by concluding that removal posed greater health risks than just leaving the material in place. The study claimed that low level exposure to chrysotile fibers, the fiber in most structures, caused few health risks compared to other fibers. Concern was expressed about the health of the workers hired to remove the substance (Times-Post News Service, 1990).

Because asbestos is rarely used alone, it is usually safe when combined with other materials as strong bonding agents. But even in well-bonded materials, asbestos can become airborne when materials are cut, sanded, or removed.

To determine if there is an asbestos problem, the only safe way is to have a sample of the material analyzed by a reliable testing company or state health agency. Since asbestos removal is hazardous, it should be done only by a qualified abatement contractor. In the process of removal, asbestos dust should not be released. It is necessary to monitor air during and after removal. Asbestos should be disposed of in a secure landfill which has been approved by the EPA.

Encapsulation is a less expensive method for control of materials which contain asbestos. It involves coating materials so that asbestos is sealed in. The process is effective only when asbestos substances are undamaged.

The best approach to asbestos removal is to become informed. One can check his home, place of work, or child's school. Asbestos may be found in such places as old ceiling tile, flaking insulation on pipes, or broken floor tile. The Better Business Bureau can recommend an asbestos removal contractor if one is needed.

Public concern has focused on the problem of asbestos in school buildings. Schools have been temporarily closed and local districts charged with enormous expenses for removal. In 1980, Congress passed the Asbestos School Hazard Detection and Removal Act to assist states and local schools in evaluating dangers and making renovations.

Research has shown that when asbestos materials age, they tend to easily crumble. Tiny particles are released into the air and can be harmful if ingested. These easily crumbled, or friable, materials were applied to overhead surfaces, walls, and pipes by spraying. It usually takes 20-25 years for building materials to deteriorate and release asbestos particles into the air.

Asbestos became especially popular in school construction because of its fireproofing, insulating, and sound absorption qualities. It was widely used in gymnasiums and auditoriums as well as classroom ceilings. Any contact, vibration, or sound can release fibers into the air. Once friable asbestos particles become airborne, they can remain in the air for months or years.

The deadline for inspecting schools and posting notices of problems was June 27, 1983. It was necessary to give each employee an EPA written guide. Results of inspection and analysis were also to be given to parent organizations such as PTO's. Officials must keep records of school inspections on hand.

Districts could have been fined for noncompliance. The emphasis was on discovering problems, formulating a plan of action, and carrying out the plan in an organized and safe manner. Besides removal, other alternatives were encapsulation and enclosure, both of which had their own drawbacks and future risks (OEA, 1983, 10-12, 20).

Dump sites in the United States may contain significant amounts of asbestos fibers. These fibers could leach so that asbestos fibers migrate into underground water. Asbestos should be discarded in licensed hazardous waste disposal sites. These sites, designed for permanent containment, should be monitored and cleaned up if public health is threatened. Wells at landfills are now being used to monitor the ground water (Peters and Peters, 1980, A 21-A 22).

There are 200,000 miles of asbestos-cement pipe in the United States. In the world, there is a total of 1,500,000 miles of such pipe. Asbestos-cement pipe was first used because of its low cost, light weight, and resistance to corrosion. In 1979, one third of all water pipe installed in the world was asbestos-cement pipe. The pipes were also used for sewers, storm drains, telephone ducts, and air ducts.

There is controversy as to whether or not asbestos fibers can be released from the pipes into the drinking water and thus end up in gastrointestinal tracts of persons. If this happens, it would be difficult to determine a specific organ in the body where the fibers may have lodged, and there would be a latency period before disease (Peters and Peters, 1980, A 18-A 19).

A decade after asbestos was identified as a powerful carcinogen, the federal government finally banned nearly all uses of the fiber with an announcement by EPA administrator William K. Reilly in July of 1989. The ban, which was first proposed in 1986, was delayed by then President Reagan's budget office. Beginning in 1990 and ending in 1997, the ban will take effect in stages.

The EPA ruling will ban the manufacture, use, and export of most asbestos products. This action is an effort to eliminate a known carcinogen from the marketplace. It will affect an estimated 94 percent of asbestos products in the United States including brake linings, roofing, pipe, tile, and insulation. The timing of the ban on certain products was based on potential human exposure and whether or not substitutes were available.

The first stage took effect in August of 1990, and applied to 10 percent of current production including roofing and flooring felt, sheeting and tile, and asbestos clothing. The second stage occurred in 1993, and affected 18 percent of products such as brake drum linings, transmission components, clutch facings, and other friction products and gaskets. The final stage, in 1996, would affect 66 percent of the asbestos market and would ban production of roof coatings, paper, brake blocks, pipes, and shingles.

The cost of the ban for industry to substitute other materials will probably be passed on to the consumer. The most far-reaching effect will be the auto industry, which had to find an alternative material for engine gaskets by 1993 and had to redesign brakes by the 1994 model year.

EPA administrator Reilly said that the 6 percent of asbestos products, which would remain on the market, pose very few health risks. Use of asbestos in the U.S. would drop to 6,000 tons by 1996.

There are many substitutes available for products formerly made from asbestos. Flame retardant suits can be made from a neoprene coated nylon fabric. Another knitted fabric can replace asbestos gloves. Asbestos roofs can be replaced with asphalt coated fiberglass ply felt. An alternative for asbestos-cement pipes are ones made with polyvinyl core wrapped with a fiber glass bonded to the core with epoxy resin. Other commonly used substitutes are fiberglass, silica fibers, ceramic fibers, mineral wool, rock wool, mica, and various plastic fibers (Peters and Peters, 1980, C 8-C 15).

In recent years, many changes regarding asbestos regulations have occurred. Numerous agencies have been involved in asbestos standards. The public has become aware that asbestos is a potential problem for everyone. Asbestos companies are paying for their past deeds. Some have changed their company names or have relegated the asbestos portion of manufacturing to a distant corner. For the most part, companies are no longer able to use the excuse that they lacked knowledge and awareness about asbestos disease. Because of asbestos companies, standards of regulation were delayed. Removal of the material from public buildings has been a costly and complicated undertaking. After an entire century of exposure abuse and resulting disease, the ban on nearly all asbestos products has finally occurred.

Chapter 23
Lacking Effective Treatment

Scientists think that all cancer begins from a single cell which divides abnormally. Abnormal growth continues in an uncontrolled manner, as the body's normal defenses are unable to stop it. Eventually, the abnormal cells form a tumor. The tumor grows between the layers of tissue, and gradually overtakes the tissue. Some cancer cells divide very quickly. Others require months or years to become visible as a tumor on an X-ray.

A malignant tumor surrounds healthy cells. Cancer cells then spread, or metastasize, to other places in the body by way of the blood system or lymph system. The original site of tumor is called the primary tumor, and secondary tumors are called metastases. If the metastases involve other organs and locations in the body, removal of the cancerous tissue and treatment of the disease is more difficult.

Treatment for mesothelioma has not been uniformly effective. Because the tumors seed themselves throughout the chest, surgical removal is not possible. In some instances, radiation has prolonged a patient's life. Radiation can be helpful, not in arresting disease, but in controlling pain and pleural effusions. The pain comes from tumor growth in sensitive nerve areas.

After daily radiation was completed and Dad had recovered some strength, he resumed outside activities. He taught his adult Sunday Sschool class and presided over deacon meetings. Mom and he traveled with the county retired teachers on an eight hour bus trip to Nashville, Tennessee, and walked around Opryland, U.S.A., not missing a step. Dad attended homecoming at the Pleasant Valley Church of the Brethren in Indiana where he spoke about the activities of each family member.

Two weeks after radiation, Dad had a follow-up appointment with the oncologist. His walking pace was slower, and he tired easily. Unless he sat a certain way, his chest ached. We applied ointment to the sore skin on his chest. With light exercise, Dad was not experiencing breathing problems. And he still had the notion that pain pills were unnecessary.

During this time, Dad participated in interviews with asbestos investigators from the Holland firm and from the affiliate law firm in South Carolina. The investigators were searching for information about asbestos products and probing Dad's mind for details about the work environment. Dad cooperated by writing answers to interrogatories and verbally describing his early memories of the foundry.

By October, his doctor appointments took place once a week, alternately with the oncologist and the chemotherapist. At Flower Hospital, Dad had regular chest X-rays and blood tests. It was still necessary to keep track of blood counts which the treatments had altered. In addition, Dad faithfully sent blood samples to the Tumor Institute in Seattle, as a follow-up to the research protocol.

The plan was that Dad would return to Seattle for a re-scanning around Thanksgiving. This trip would provide an opportunity to schedule a permanent nerve block on Dad's chest. When the nerves frozen during surgery began to grow, a more permanent nerve block could alleviate further discomfort.

Mom and Dad bought their plane tickets for the November trip. They planned to arrive before Thanksgiving and stay about a week, allowing time for the holiday and for consultation with doctors.

By the last week in October, Dad's social schedule became more than he could tolerate. We worried about the threat of germs attacking his weakened body. When his temperature fluctuated from morning to evening, and he developed a cough, we were concerned that he had pneumonia. Dad became so weak that Mom finally took him to the Bryan Medical Center. Since the doctor there was unfamiliar with Dad's case, he called Flower Hospital for advice. Dad got an appointment for the next day at Flower. As the higher temperature was not a constant thing, the local doctor thought Dad didn't have pneumonia. A meeting with the chemotherapist was planned for the first week in November.

I was involved in teaching and new school year activities such as open house and parent-teacher conferences. Since school had started, I usually only accompanied Dad when his appointments were in the late afternoon. I regretted not paying closer attention.

At the November 2 meeting, the chemotherapist explained a new regimen of treatment. The agent this time would be Adriamycin. A couple months earlier, the oncologist had told us that Adriamycin did not have a proven success rate, though in some types of cancer, it had been helpful. Information about its use with mesothelioma was incomplete.

The chemotherapist felt that Dad was strong enough and his mesothelioma insidious enough that Adriamycin could be given intravenously every three weeks. Even though we had been concerned about pneumonia the week before, Dad was willing to try additional chemotherapy.

The reaction, or side effects, to Adriamycin would be more noticeable than the cisplatinum had been. Like platinum, Adriamycin could cause kidney and bladder problems. Other side effects to expect were an irregular heartbeat, swelling of the legs and feet, chills, and fever, all requiring medical attention. One definite side effect would be the loss of hair. Since Dad rarely threw up, nausea would be less of a problem. Each patient reacts individually to the medication.

Dad was determined to keep fighting the cancer. He did not intend to give in to it. In retrospect, the beginning of this chemotherapy regimen started Dad's decline. He was already experiencing a weakened state. Fibrosis of his right lung from radiation and the resulting accumulation of fluids was building up. It strained his body and his breathing.

I had thought everything was going satisfactorily. Raising the question that maybe Dad couldn't tolerate more chemotherapy didn't occur to me. The treatments were characteristically debilitating. Wasn't that the price for killing off cancer cells? It was hard to separate the side effects of chemotherapy from the symptoms of disease to determine his real condition.

A week after the first treatment, all of Dad's hair fell out. I had thought this would be a gradual loss. Dad's chemotherapy dosage had been based on his age and weight, but the medication had produced severe effects. The following week, his blood counts plummeted to a dangerously low level. His white blood count, the protection against germs, which normally should range from 4 to 10, fell to .6. His platelet count was 82,000, when a normal range is 150,000 to 400,000.

The extreme drop in counts really frightened us, and we called Flower Hospital. They requested that Bryan retest his blood the following day to see if the counts were rising. The next blood test revealed a white blood count of .9, and a platelet count of 131,000, which indicated that the figures were improving. It was suggested that Dad be retested in two or three days. Not only was Dad weak and susceptible to infection, he was giving vial after vial of blood for analysis.

Because of this development, Dad's health was deemed too unsteady to risk the flight to Seattle. Another set of plans had to be canceled. The trip wouldn't be worth the effort if Dad's health would be further jeopardized by the journey.

It was a deep disappointment that my parents had to alter their plans. Not only had Dad lost his hair, but now he was primarily housebound. And his chest pain was increasing. How and when would he get the needed nerve block? I wondered.

Within three days, Dad's blood counts had again reached acceptable levels. Mom and he went to a Thanksgiving dinner sponsored by GALA, a county program for senior citizens. That dinner was Dad's last social outing. Future outings would mostly be trips to the doctor or hospital.

Dad was timid about the loss of his hair. Mom was concerned about his loss of body heat in the cold, winter weather. Within two days, Dad agreed to meet with a woman who specialized in wigs for cancer patients. During his visit, she styled a brown wig with a full head of hair for Dad. He looked about thirty years younger. The wig not only provided warmth, but it was very becoming on him.

Another post-chemotherapy occurrence was body temperature variation. In the evenings, Dad's fever would rise. During the night, he sweated heavily and had to change his bed clothes. Next, he experienced violent chills. In the morning, his temperature dropped below normal. Doctors had not predicted this symptom. Was it related to the chemo and should we be concerned? Dad began to carry a thermometer, taking his temperature at intervals and keeping a chart of the results. His temperature varied widely, but the pattern was consistent. We didn't know what it meant.

For the late November chemotherapy, the dosage of Adriamycin was lowered. The oncology nurse said it was more important to avoid a break in treatment by lowering the dosage than to skip a treatment. That way, chemo would work continuously in the body.

A friend of mine, who had been a cancer patient, once told me that she was not concerned about enduring chemotherapy, as toxic and energy-sapping as it was. What worried her most was the end of treatments. During chemo, she knew the cancer cells were being arrested. But after the chemo regimen was over, she was unsure about what the cancer cells were doing.

I think my father, too, welcomed another round of chemotherapy. Even though he disliked the process, submitting to treatment meant that his doctors and he were still attacking the disease. It didn't occur to us that the doctor's decision for further treatment indicated that the cancer was progressing.

Chemotherapy, or treating cancer with drugs, was first done in 1945. New drugs for cancer were discovered in the fifties and sixties for use with previously incurable cancers. Even though thousands of chemical agents are tested each year, very few make it into experimental cancer programs after the laboratory and animal testing is done. Instead, researchers work on combining current drugs into more effective variations. The main problems are still the undesirable side effects and the damage caused to normal cells.

In the past decade, the newest cancer treatments have involved stimulating the body's own immune system to control the growth of cancer cells. This process, known as immunotherapy, assumes that if one's immune system is stimulated, it can reject or attack cancer cells. The technology of producing immune-cell products outside the body makes immunotherapy possible (Johnson and Klein, 1988, 59). Substances such as interferon, interleukin-2, and monoclonal antibodies are examples of such biological modifiers which can be injected in the body.

Interferon and interleukin-2 are two recent forms of treatment. Interferon, a family of proteins, is naturally produced by the body in response to viral infections. It was named because it interferes with the reproduction of viruses. Its presence in the body was discovered in 1957, but it was not manufactured in the lab for practical use until 1981. Interferon has been effective in fighting a few cancers, and has had moderate success with others. Its use has not had the widespread success originally predicted with more common forms such as breast, lung, or colon cancers. Interleukin-2 is cultured in a test tube with a patient's white blood cells. The culture is then injected in the body, along with pure interleukin-2. In use since 1986, the method has been used with metastatic cancers, but it is complicated, toxic, and costly.

As I read about new cancer treatments, I became particularly interested in monoclonal antibodies. The idea that antibodies can be produced and programmed to attack specific cancer cells sounded revolutionary. Monoclonal antibodies are antibodies produced from a single line, or clone. The procedure is similar to that used in vaccinations for disease. In the method, the antigens from a patient's cancer cells are injected into laboratory animals. As a result, the animals produce antibodies to that particular kind of cancer. The antibodies are then removed from the animal and mixed with a patient's own white blood cells to which the antibodies bind. The substance, now with unlimited antibodies, is injected into the patient. The antibodies assist in marking tumor cells for destruction (Johnson and Klein, 1988, 37-38).

Monoclonal antibodies were first produced in 1979, and used in clinical trials. About 200 such antibodies have been produced in the lab. The first use of monoclonal antibodies, along with radioactive isotopes to scan the body for cancer cells, was in 1983. Their major use has been in diagnosis, although they have been effective in treating cancers such as leukemia and lymphoma (Goldberg, 1988, 17-18).

In the future, persons may be tested to find out if they lack certain proteins and enzymes in the immune system. Dosages of the missing substances could be given. There might also be anti-cancer vaccines and monoclonal antibody infusions given to individuals determined to be at risk. More attention is being paid to anti-cancer lifestyles which include a low-fat, high-fiber diet, psychological well-being, and avoidance of exposure to carcinogens (Dreher, 1988, 32-33).

Unfortunately, an antibody for my father's cancer has not yet been found. Dad was hopeful about a new treatment in three or four years. During the course of his illness, he mentioned that possibility to several doctors.

In late November, two childhood friends of Dad's from Indiana stopped one evening for a visit. Mom and I attended a Christmas concert, but Dad did not feel like going. Upon our return, Dad was busily chatting with Bill and Miriam Cable. Dad proudly showed off his new wig. The Cables marveled at Dad's bright spirit and positive outlook. They had previously inquired about Dad's condition, and they knew he had been through debilitating treatments. With the Cables, we formed a prayer circle to ask for God's influence in Dad's illness. Afterwards, the Cables continued to provide support via phone calls and daily prayers.

During the holidays, Dad was serenaded by our church's annual Christmas caroling party. Usually, the carolers stop at the homes of shut-ins. This year, Dad qualified as a recipient of this ministry. He humbly stood in the doorway as the traditional melodies filled the air. The singing brought tears to his eyes.

We held the usual Christmas celebrations in which Dad took part without complaint. Even though he couldn't attend church functions, he went to family gatherings. He received his share of neck mufflers and self-help books.

Milan's family arrived a few days after Christmas. By this time, Dad's chest pain caused him to walk in a stooped over position. His clothes hung loosely on him, and his smile for photographs hid the pain. He could sit only a little while and would take frequent rest breaks. However, the joy of having family members home brightened his countenance. Indeed, his outward glow surpassed the inward havoc of the cancer cells.

Chapter 24
Nearing the End of the Struggle

On the first official day of winter, Dad received his third Adria-mycin treatment. It was not the best timing for beginning the holiday week, since side effects would appear between Christmas and New Year's Day. Because the wind chill registered sixty degrees below zero, we enlisted a young man from church to drive to Flower Hospital. They encountered no problems during the trip. Wind chills plummeted even further the next day.

During the fall, I myself had been plagued with recurring colds and fever. The demanding days of teaching wore me down. Dad's progressively worsening condition concerned me, including the fear that he might contract pneumonia. My empathy grew so strong that I decided I must have pneumonia, too. My doctor arranged a chest X-ray and prescribed stronger medication. The doctor ruled out anything serious.

On Christmas Eve, a dear lady in our church suffered a heart attack. She lingered near death in the local hospital's intensive care unit. For a week, her children, grandchildren, and great-grandchildren spoke with her and said good-bye. As a result, the holiday season was very strenuous for them. The woman died on January 2. My father insisted on visiting the funeral home to pay his respects. Despite several years of heart problems, the woman had been an influential and active member of the congregation. As I attended her funeral, I watched the devastated family members. The congregation recited the Twenty-third Psalm by memory. How soon would such an event occur in my family? I wondered.

It was near the end of the school's first semester. My students would have a vacation on Martin Luther King, Jr. Day while we teachers averaged semester grades. I envied their break. I told my co-teacher that I didn't know how much longer I could continue my teaching duties when I was so concerned about my father.

On January 11, 1990, Dad went to the hospital for his fourth

Adriamycin chemotherapy. My parents' friend, Vernon Grim, accompanied them. The treatment was planned for morning, and typically, they would have returned home by late afternoon. Sleet was falling outside when I called my parents and got no answer. By early evening, I phoned Mrs. Grim to find out if she had heard from them. I felt like the mother of teen-agers trying to locate offspring who are out beyond curfew.

Shortly afterwards, Mom called to tell me that Dad had been admitted to Flower Hospital. The oncology nurses had noted Dad's condition before treatment and advised that he be admitted. Not only were his blood counts low, but he had pneumonia as well. We had been concerned about Dad's weakened condition, his temperature variations, his blood test results, and his constant cough. His contracting pneumonia was our worst fear, and we hadn't been able to prevent it.

Because I did not want to act unduly alarmed, I continued teaching. I went to the hospital on weekends, while my mother made daily trips. Dad was assigned to a private room on the seventh floor. His room was designed for comfort and healing since it resembled a deluxe hotel room with plush carpet, fancy curtains, elegant wallpaper, and two phones. Evening snacks were available, and family members could sleep on the couch overnight.

A couple days stretched into a week and then two weeks. Every four hours, Dad received breathing treatments on a pulmonary machine. Because of his weakness, he was mostly bedridden. He had a variety of doctors including a lung specialist, a nerve specialist, a radiologist, his regular chemotherapist, and the oncologist. The doctors conversed with Dad on their early morning and late evening rounds. Since Mom and I were not at the hospital at those hours, we were not in close contact with the doctors. They had determined that the pneumonia was in the damaged lung and the pain was partly caused by fibrosis due to radiation.

Because of Dad's chest pain, an anesthesiologist attempted a nerve block. Dad had been hoping for this procedure. Using needles around the chest, the doctor tried several temporary blocks. It was a disappointment that the nerve blocks did not ease the pain.

One day, an ice storm kept us home from the hospital. When we went the following day, Dad was in an agitated state. He had refused his dinner, his pain medication, and his physical therapy. When we questioned the nurses, they replied that Dad had been uncooperative. Further discussion revealed that the pain medication had caused him constipation. In his frantic state, he was unable to convey the message to staff. We were unhappy with Dad's behavior and uncomfortable that such lack of communication would occur in our absence.

After viewing Dad's X-rays, the doctors told us that his right lung had mostly collapsed. The radiation and fluid build-up pressure, along with the pneumonia, had demanded too much. Instead of releasing Dad, the radiologist decided to perform a bronchoscopy. The bronchoscopy, a direct examination of the lungs, reminded Dad of surgery and distressed him.

Our minister arrived to visit Dad, and she remarked that the elevator doors had opened immediately and brought her to the seventh floor. I told her it was a sign that she was urgently needed. Dad clutched the minister's hand as tears welled up in his eyes. Mom worried about the pneumonia spreading to the other lung. We held hands and prayed for Dad's strength.

In a bronchoscopy, the air passages of the lungs are examined using a flexible tube with a light attached to it. Medication beforehand relaxes the patient and dries up secretions. During the procedure, specimens are taken and air passages washed out. The radiologist inserts a tube through the nose or mouth down to the trachea and bronchi, without blocking the airways. Gagging may occur initially, and then subside. The actual procedure takes from thirty to sixty minutes. The only aftereffects are a sore throat and numbness (Pramik, 1985). The radiologist took cultures from both lungs for further study.

At some point, we knew Dad would have difficulty with his right lung. Radiation had constantly bombarded the lung, and the plugged mucous was bound to cause problems. Hopefully, it had been advantageous to clean out the secretions so they would not continue to breed bacteria. After the bronchoscopy, the lung doctor told us that the right lung would not get much better. I reminded Mom that we had expected to sacrifice one lung in hopes of eradicating the cancer.

Besides receiving oxygen through a tube in his nose, another positive result of Dad's January hospitalization was acquiring a TENS unit to relieve pain. TENS is an abbreviation for transcutaneous electric nerve stimulation. The unit resembles a transistor radio and operates by battery power. The unit itself is clipped to a cuff or pocket. Electrodes are attached to pads which are spaced apart and placed on the skin. Flexible wires connect the electrodes to the box-like unit. In order to block the body's own pain signals to the brain, electrical impulses are generated from the box to nerve endings (Anderson, 1990, 1185). The location of the chest pads had to be changed about every third day to avoid burning the skin. Power from a C-size battery is exhausted every other day.

We soon learned how to change the pads and regulate the controls. We turned the dials until Dad experienced a tingling feeling. The hospital loaned the use of the TENS unit for thirty days, after which we would need to purchase a unit from a pharmacy for about $1,000. The handy unit was the first relief from pain Dad had encountered. Soon, he no longer had to be convinced to use the unit consistently.

One of Dad's male nurses closely resembled a professional football player, since he was 6'7" and weighed about 250 pounds. When Dad asked him why he had become a nurse instead of a doctor, the male nurse replied that he wanted time to spend his money. Every eight hours, the nursing staff changed; and each day, nurses rotated to various floors. Different pulmonary therapists assisted Dad every day. Dad took the influx of staff cheerfully.

Dad worked hard to regain his strength. By the second and third week, he went to physical therapy twice a day on the ground floor of the hospital. A therapist pushed him by wheelchair, using elevators for patients only. If Dad was eating or visiting with company, the schedule was flexible.

In therapy, the therapist involved Dad in several exercises. He used a walker in a circular path around the ward. He raised a wooden cane with weights attached, similar to a barbell. He lifted his legs from the hip and knee. He strengthened his legs by placing weights on his ankles and doing leg lifts.

When Dad's hospital stay extended, get well cards began to arrive. He treasured each card and handwritten note. Dad was part of our local church's prayer chain and was included in prayer chains from Harrisburg, Pennsylvania, to Denver, Colorado. We appreciated such warm wishes of support. Since Dad's phone was attached to his bed, he easily received phone calls from concerned friends. All the messages, both written and verbal, had a positive effect.

Dad knew he would be released from the hospital when the director of social services visited his room. Dad said we should meet with her to make arrangements. He repeatedly reminded us.

By the third week, I took days off school to help make plans. I tried to think of contacts we needed to make before Dad came home. Because Dad required extensive care, I felt Mom needed relief from cooking. Thus, I suggested a program of home-delivered meals. We wondered if Dad would still need an artificial oxygen supply. We wanted him to continue the physical therapy exercises. We considered the therapy equipment needed as well as a walker and cane, a bedside commode, and a bench for the bathtub. I wondered how we would keep track of Dad's condition without nursing care. A nurse could also come to take his blood samples. Making these contacts seemed overwhelming.

Fortunately, the experienced social services director had thought of these issues, too. She knew specific contacts to make in our county. Her knowledge relieved our stress as she anticipated our needs. She arranged for the local home health agency to visit my parents' home for an initial evaluation and interview.

On the morning of his release, Dad awoke while it was still dark outside. His actual release was still tentative, but not to him. Dad later claimed he had misread the clock. After midnight, Dad got up, unassisted, and dressed in the suit he had worn during admission. Just to be prepared, he also put on his overcoat and hat. When he realized his mistake, he lay back down on the bed and fell asleep. The amused staff must have wondered how Dad had accomplished the task by himself. I could have told them it was sheer determination! When the staff checked during the night, he was fast asleep on the bed, fully clothed, and grasping his cane as if ready to walk out.

By midday, Dad's release papers, his list of instructions from doctors, and his prescription bottles were ready. Dad rode a wheelchair to the car. When he reached home, however, he had to be carried in, as he was unaccustomed to being upright for a length of time.

The kitchen counter resembled a mini-pharmacy. Among the medicines were pain pills, Tylenol, antibiotics, vitamins, iron pills, constipation medicine, and Bumex, or water pills. Dad still hesitated to take pain medicine. Part of his aversion to such medicine was that his mother had suffered kidney damage as a result of taking too much pain medicine for migraine headaches.

Dad disliked the "water pill" the most. Its purpose was to relieve the swelling in his legs and ankles. An unpleasant side effect was a run to the bathroom every few minutes for about four hours. Dad had difficulty with mobility, and this presented an added burden.

The interview with the home health agency director lasted three hours. In addition to meeting us, she assessed Dad's condition and explained the procedures of the agency. She scheduled visits by a registered nurse twice a week and a nursing aid on other days. She said that the agency can be called at any time of the day or night for medical help. Besides monitoring Dad's physical condition, the nurses would change the TENS unit pads, check medications, and assist Dad in bathing and getting dressed.

In her written report, the director noted Dad's slightly diminished heart volume and elevated pulse. She listed fatigue, poor appetite, and shortness of breath. Of the greatest concern was his low blood pressure which was 62/40. The water pills were the probable cause, yet she could not alter medication without the doctor's permission. She called Flower Hospital, and the water pill intake was changed to every other day. I was glad we had a knowledgeable person as an intercessory. At the end of her report, she included how attentive we were to Dad and what an excellent understanding of the disease we had.

In two days, Dad's blood pressure returned to normal, and his heart volume grew stronger. His appetite improved, and he became more alert. Because of his unsteady balance and slow gait, he gingerly used a pronged cane. He had a nonproductive cough and an irregular respiration. Edema, or swelling, was present in both lower legs and ankles, and the nurse instructed him to wear loose slippers and avoid salt intake. Dad demonstrated his therapy exercises, and the nurse suggested he keep track of the number done.

Dad spent most of the day sitting in his favorite reclining chair. He positioned a box of Kleenex and wastebasket on one side and a glass of juice on the other. Coughing was a constant companion, and he strained to make the cough productive. Dad fell in and out of sleep, and several times a day, he would exercise and rest.

By the first of February, Dad's heart volume was strong, but its rhythm slightly irregular. Dad complained that his back and side were painful, even when sitting upright. Dad began to describe a floating feeling which he said was like rolling on gentle waves. The floating feeling impaired his reading ability and sense of balance.

We were extremely concerned about Dad's exposure to unwanted germs. If someone came for a visit, we quizzed them about their physical condition before letting them enter. We were still hoping Dad would improve. The Adriamycin chemotherapy had ended with Dad's January hospitalization. Instead of helping, the treatments had further weakened him.

By February 5, Dad's total weight loss since the surgery was thirty to thirty-five pounds. The home health nurse suggested that Dad eat smaller, more frequent meals of high calorie foods. We purchased numerous flavors of a liquid nutrient for Dad to drink. Even with the TENS unit and the pain pills, Dad experienced pain. He became short of breath when ambulatory.

Mom brought Dad's meals to him on a tray. Since Dad had so little control over his circumstances, he gave detailed directions about what he wanted. I knew he did this in frustration, yet this habit was irritating.

Before Dad's post-hospital checkup, he was exercising hard. Instead of using his cane, he carried it in his arms. When I assisted him with therapy, we discussed how he would hopefully get stronger while his remaining lung gradually compensated. I wondered if Dad overdid the exercise routine. He lifted weights until he had to gasp for breath. I wanted Dad to enjoy some normal activity soon. Someday, we hoped to schedule a more permanent nerve block.

At his follow-up appointment with the oncologist, Dad's blood count was fairly good. There were no major changes in his condition. The doctor told him to breathe deeply and to stay away from colds and infections.

Two days later, Mom called the home health nurse because of Dad's shortness of breath and the swelling in his legs. The nurse made an unscheduled visit and found Dad's pulse elevated to 140 and his heart rhythm irregular. Both sides of his legs and feet had edema. The nurse called the doctor who instructed Dad to take his water pills and pain pills. The second session of the caregiving seminar with Rev. Flinchbaugh was held the same day, and Dad was unable to go.

Within two days, we consulted an anesthesiologist at Flower Hospital regarding a nerve block. Dad explained his intercostal nerve block with liquid nitrogen which the surgeon had done. The anesthesiologist said he could do a temporary nerve block which would last six to twelve months. Special equipment was needed for a more permanent one. He checked with Toledo Hospital, the Medical College of Ohio, and with hospitals in Detroit and Cleveland to find out if one could be arranged. While we waited, the doctor was unable to make phone contacts. Thus, we accomplished nothing that day, and a nerve block seemed like an ever illusive event.

On February 14, which was my parents' forty-seventh wedding anniversary, Vernon Grim drove them to an appointment with the lung specialist at the Toledo Clinic. I carefully wrote out directions to the clinic and a list of questions to ask. Mom asked the doctor if Dad's feeling of motion and his fast breathing rate were caused by a lack of oxygen. The doctor said that Dad's weakened shape and fluctuating blood pressure could be contributing factors. Water retention caused the swelling in his legs and feet. Dad was coping as well as could be expected. The receptionist arranged a nerve block for February 22.

Mom and I spent a Saturday at a stage play in Toledo. Dad balked at our leaving for the afternoon. We invited a friend from church to keep Dad company. Dad talked with his visitor until he was hoarse.

The next day, Dad experienced spells when he totally lost his energy. He had to lie down in exhaustion while his heart pounded. In the afternoon, I told a friend that I didn't know what to do. I knew Dad preferred not to return to the hospital. Mom and I would wait to see what developed. However, as sometimes happens, events progressed beyond our control.

Ironically, the home health nurse arrived unexpectedly the following day, Presidents' Day. Upon examination, she noted Dad's extreme shortness of breath and apparent weakness. She called Flower Hospital to check if Dad should be admitted. The doctor returned the call and said to bring Dad in. I expected Dad to stubbornly refuse this pronouncement, and I prepared to argue the inevitable with him.

Early in the week, Ohio had endured two successive days of sleet. The first storm had iced over the roads and trees and forced officials to cancel school. The second onslaught added another layer to already burdened tree branches. Nearly every tree suffered damage, and broken twigs and branches lay in heaps on the ground. My parents' yard was hit hard. I didn't know how we would clear away such a mess.

When I arrived, a pickup truck and two cars with open trunks were backed into the driveway. Three men from our church were using chain saws to cut wood and load it into vehicles. The sight of their work moved me to tears. All three had attended the caregiving seminar. I remembered that one had wondered how he could be helpful in a practical way. These men had found a way to lend assistance. As they moved about the yard sawing off branches and gathering wood, they illustrated caregivers in action. My father watched them from the window. These generous men were attending to one of our problems, while we faced an even larger one.

Chapter 25
Requiring Rehospitalization

As I entered the house, Dad was sitting in the den with the nurse's aid at his side. Getting ready to return to the hospital had required much physical effort. Each time a spell of breathlessness overcame him, Dad had to stop and rest. Mom was at loose ends deciding what to pack. Convincing Dad to go had not been a problem, but getting organized and mentally prepared was a challenge. Dad had been home for only three weeks. He had put forth valiant effort and had looked forward to springlike weather when he could go outside. Now, we would trace our familiar path to Flower Hospital.

Because of his lack of strength, we carried Dad to the car. As I drove, I glanced at Dad's drawn and weak face in the rear view mirror. He had come on this trip without complaint or questions. Our plan of Dad becoming stronger and having a period free from disease was not occurring. It was difficult for me to change from positive hopes for Dad to witnessing his physical chore to just stay alive.

It was after 5 P.M. when we pulled up to the hospital entrance. Windy, cold air greeted us as we transferred Dad from the back seat to the wheelchair. While I parked the car, Mom pushed Dad to the registration area. When the receptionist assigned Dad to the third floor, we said that he had previously been in a private room on the seventh floor. She placed another call and then escorted us to the seventh floor.

We were unpacking Dad's things as a nurse went through a list of questions with Dad. Then, the lung doctor came in. In an exasperated manner, he asked what we were doing on the seventh floor. We replied that we thought Dad had been assigned here. The doctor further scolded us for being late. I tried to explain the distance we had driven and the difficulty of getting Dad ready. Mom said that we just wanted Dad to be on the floor where he would get the best care.

The doctor motioned Mom and me to the hallway. He then explained that heart patients were assigned to the third floor so they could be more closely monitored. Why would Dad be a heart patient? I wondered. We still had no idea what was wrong. The doctor said that the tumors had probably surrounded Dad's heart, and we would need to decide soon whether or not we wanted the staff to use resuscitation on him and what kind. My mouth shuddered.

The doctor wondered if anyone had discussed the disease with us. I replied that we knew about the disease, but we didn't realize that it now involved Dad's heart. But pneumonia had severely weakened Dad. Now, he would need to be moved to the coronary floor to be monitored. How did the doctor know this before examining Dad? I asked myself. Tears streamed down my face as I returned to take Dad's things from the closet for his move to the coronary floor.

His room was located directly across from the nurses' station. A curtain separated his bed from his roommate. I wondered how he would be able to make it back and forth to the bathroom. While we waited, a nurse took Dad's vital statistics, and a young man did an EKG. One of the nurses apologized for the moving around we had done.

While Dad ate, I went to the telephones by the elevators. It was time to let my brothers know Dad was back in the hospital. I dreaded making the calls. I had hoped such calls would be months or years away. I didn't want to think about resuscitation, but what if Dad had difficulty and we hadn't decided how to respond? Why had it all been reduced to this? Didn't any of the treatments make a difference? I wasn't ready to face my father's death. I had just brought him to the hospital where he had gotten better before. I wanted to call my brothers so they would have an opportunity to come to Ohio while Dad was still able to talk with them.

I first placed a call to my brother, Dean. His wife, Mary, answered, and all I was able to say was that Dad was back in the hospital, and I burst out crying. Mary had recognized my voice and responded calmly. At the time, Dean was out. She said she knew it was difficult, and I had been under a lot of pressure. If I just said the word, Dean would be on a plane that night. Mary said we had done the right thing by bringing Dad to the hospital where he could get proper care.

When I could finally speak, I said that I didn't always know what to do. The doctors wanted to know what methods of resuscitation we were requesting, and I hadn't even known there were different levels. Mary said that we had known this day would come, but I questioned why it had come so soon. She said Dean would call the hospital as soon as he got in.

I swallowed, took a deep breath, and called Milan's number. Milan answered immediately. I said that Dad was back in the hospital, and the doctor thought the tumors were around his heart. I thought he would like to know, in case he wanted to come. And I asked him what he thought about the resuscitation.

Milan had trouble hearing me, and I had to repeat the information. He said he had planned to leave on a business trip the next day, and might have to make other arrangements. In case he couldn't change his plans, he gave me the numbers where he could be reached.

Mom came into the waiting area and wondered who I was talking with. I handed her the phone. Mom told Milan that coming should be his decision, and might not be absolutely necessary at this point. Her own denial was apparent. I felt relieved that I had relayed the news to both my brothers.

Mom and I stayed at the hospital until about 11 P.M., and Dad seemed to be settling in. Since I had school the next morning, we decided to leave for home. Mom and I were both exhausted, and Dad thought he could get along until morning. We kissed him good-night. Mom planned to return in the morning, and I would come later in the day.

It was after midnight when I got home. It still did not occur to me to take the next day off school. I didn't want to admit that the time had come. Dean called and asked how things were going. He had checked on Dad by calling the nurses' station. He said that the resuscitation question was routine for patients such as Dad. Dean said he would discuss the possibilities with Mom, and I should get some rest. He also said he would let me know his plans for coming to Ohio.

After an hour, my bedside phone rang. I had not been sleeping anyway, and I anxiously picked up the receiver. It was a nurse in Flower Hospital's Intensive Care Unit (ICU). She had tried to reach my mother and had gotten no answer. Dad's heart rate had escalated to the point that they had transferred him to intensive care. They would try to get the rate down and watch him closely. I asked her if we should come back to the hospital, and she said to hold off, for the time being. She had called because it was their policy to let families know when patients had been moved to ICU. I said that I would relay the message and that we would come in the morning. Since my mother was exhausted, I decided to share the news with her the next day.

I dialed Dean, who fortunately was in the Pacific time zone where it was three hours earlier. I told him about Dad, and he said he would call the hospital to find out more details. It was 3s A.M. as I waited wide-eyed for his return call. I could never make it to school now, I thought, and I might not sleep at all. There were too many adjustments to make in this developing situation. I thought about what Dad had been through to fight the cancer and how unfair this seemed. I just hoped that he survived the night.

Dean called to say that Dad's heart rate had risen to over 200 beats per minute. With medication and IVs, the rate was going down, but was still elevated. I thought it had been bad enough to worry about the cancer, and now we had to be concerned about Dad's heart rate. When I hung up, I could picture the tumors moving in around Dad's heart. As long as I was awake, maybe Dad could keep going, too. During the rest of the night, I grieved for the impending loss of my father.

Chapter 26
Receiving Coronary Care

After his move to ICU, Dad survived the night. His heart rate was near 170, and he was on a fast heart drip. The medicine was an attempt to keep the rate under control. Earlier, Dad had been coughing and felt as if something was caught in his throat. Amazingly, because the fast heart rate exhausted him, he had slept much of the night. Mom told the nurse that her sons lived quite a distance away, but the nurse said not to call them home unless they would normally visit. She added that the ICU staff was working to keep the heart rate down, and a heart specialist had been called to examine Dad.

Meanwhile, Dean called to tell me Milan would fly in that afternoon, and I should meet him at the Toledo airport. Dean said he would try to come later in the week. Milan had been at the Philadelphia airport trying to decide whether to go on his business trip to South Carolina or to come to Ohio. For awhile, he had purchased tickets for both destinations. Then, he was able to delay his business meetings and board the Ohio bound plane.

When we arrived at ICU on the hospital's first floor, our minister was already talking with Dad. As we entered, Dad greeted us with a smile. He was hooked up to various IVs and machines.

Before we had time to talk, a therapist came to do a heart sonogram and invited us to watch the procedure. She rubbed lotion on Dad's chest, and then moved a probe scan around the heart area. As she did so, a picture appeared on a television monitor. She spoke into a microphone as she recorded the location of the sonogram. To me, it looked like black and gray shadows with a vibration near the center.

ICU didn't seem like a place for rest. A custodian pushed a noisy vacuum near the doorway. The nurse said that Dad was doing better. Since there was an incoming surgical patient, Dad would be transferred to the Coronary Unit, another ward on the third floor. This would make Dad's fourth move in eighteen hours. For the transfer, I thought they would disconnect some of the machines, but instead, the orderlies just placed them around the bed's framework and rolled the entire load onto a large elevator.

The Coronary Care Unit, known as CCU, was a separate section on the coronary floor. There were two parts within CCU, and entrance was limited to family members during specified times. The more ambulatory coronary patients occupied regular rooms. Dad was assigned a small, private room in an area for more critical care patients. He could be watched closely through a window which opened to a central nurses' station. A private coronary care nurse would attend him.

Shortly after his move, I left for the airport. Dad didn't question why Milan was coming so suddenly, but just seemed pleased that he would see him. When I reached the terminal, Milan had just deboarded, and I ran to hug him. He had come to help us, and would be able to stay for the rest of the week. I was grateful my brother had arrived.

During the week, we made daily trips to the hospital. When we were not at the hospital, we called the CCU nurses' station for updates. Dean usually called the nurses, and then he called us. As a physician, he could ask more knowledgeable questions. In the evenings, we called Dean with nightly reports, and our phone bills were enormous.

The CCU nurses were especially caring. They were specially trained for intensive care, and they worked twelve hour shifts, two to three times a week. They did not know how to operate the TENS unit, and initially thought that it might interfere with the heart monitor equipment. A physical therapist came to demonstrate its use for them. Just when we got to know one nurse, another would take her place. One nurse noticed the thickness of Dad's medical records and asked us about Dad's medical history.

The nurses kept a written report in a large notebook. It included medications, doctor visits, vital statistics, and even notes about family visits. Once in a while, we peeked at it when we first arrived. Dad was hooked up to five IVs. His arms were black and blue. Since he was never out of bed, he quit wearing his wig and wore a colored cap instead. During his week in CCU, he ate fairly well. We filled out menu choices of a balanced diet which included foods that were easily palatable.

Other patients moved in and out of critical care CCU, but Dad remained day after day. Above Dad, a monitor registered his heart rate, and the numbers and pattern were visible to everyone but

Dad. The numbers fluctuated from 98 to 170, often varying by the second. A wavy line showed his heart's irregular rhythm. Periodically, his heart would go into atrial fibrillation, an involuntary contraction of the atrial chamber, which disrupted the heart's normal sinus rhythm. Treatments of digitalis were administered in order to restore normal rhythm.

One of Dad's frequent questions, in concern about his rapid heart rate, was to ask if his chest was heaving up and down. Of course, one side of his chest barely moved. And the other side did not appear abnormal. We spoke to him reassuringly. The results of the recent heart sonogram did not show any damage to the heart itself. However, because of Dad's collapsed right lung, the heart muscle had stretched over to the right side. Despite this, the heart rate had been reasonably controlled with medication. Dad's internal organs were doing a delicate balancing act.

Each additional day seemed like a blessing. Dad was in a quiet, accepting mood. Our goals became more short term such as helping him eat, hoping the swelling in his legs went down, and wondering if his heart rate was relatively steady. The heart medicine lowered his blood pressure, and the respiratory medicine increased the heart rate. Doctors modified the oxygen level when needed. An unwanted weight gain from fluid retention occurred several times. Because he was so weak, Dad was placed in a hammock to be weighed. If there was fluid gain, the medication had to be altered. It was a challenge for doctors to balance one problem against the other. When we were present, Dad was awake and alert. When we were not with him, he slept. At times, the physical stress on his body caused him to be somewhat disoriented.

I decided to speak with Dad on a personal level. It was too difficult to talk about death. However, I wanted to express to Dad my appreciation for his efforts as my father. As I sat on the edge of the bed, Dad gently held my hand. I told him he had been a good father, and I had depended on him many times, even as an adult. He had been my protection, and I had needed his guidance. I knew he had worked hard to care for us. I said he had given me opportunities because of his sacrifices, and he had helped me in many practical ways. I thanked him for being a loving father. I said I was sorry he had suffered, but I was impressed with his courage in facing illness. He replied that he had always tried to teach me the right things. He had done things for his family that he wished his father had done for him.

Milan also had the opportunity to talk with Dad. They discussed Milan's old basketball games, as only they remembered them. I had been fearful that Milan would not see his father, but he spent an entire week visiting and reminiscing with him. On Saturday, we took Milan to the airport so he could return to his family.

Shortly after Milan's plane departed, a whiteout occurred. Sleet accompanied the whiteout, and we decided to start home from the hospital early. The turnpike toll booth attendant advised us that there had been numerous accidents, and the turnpike was closed to incoming traffic. The only place I could think of going was the home of a friend's mother near the exit.

We are grateful to my friend and her mother for taking us in that night. The roads were not drivable, and we were already stressed from dealing with Dad's hospitalization. They welcomed us and fed us. The next day, looking a bit bedraggled, we went again to the airport to meet my brother Dean.

Dad perked up when Dean arrived. He thought Dean would know what the situation was and could communicate it to us. We put pressure on Dean to inform us, and sometimes, we asked questions for which there were no answers. I was glad Dean had come in time to see his father.

Dad talked about the possibility of a service with our minister. The purpose of this service would be a statement of faith and prayers for spiritual wholeness. We held the service in Dad's hospital room. Not only was Dean present, but Mom's brother and his wife also participated.

My uncle had been calling from Texas each evening to find out about Dad's condition. Mom had discouraged them from leaving their winter haven. She didn't want to tell them to come home. By the end of the week, they just informed us they were coming. While pulling a forty-foot trailer, they drove to Ohio in record time. It was the same icy weekend we had been stranded in Toledo.

Dad's sister, Carolyn, came to visit Dad from Indiana. Dad and she talked about their early life together. During her visit, Dad's heart rate became elevated. Balancing his medical condition was becoming harder. Carolyn said later that losing her brother would make her the last member of her immediate family.

Dean discussed the levels of resuscitation with my mother. These included CPR, heart resuscitation, electric shock and a ventilator. Of course, the hospital staff does everything possible until the family gives more specific instructions. A ventilator is usually used for a patient's breathing when he needs to get over a hump. However, removing a ventilator can require a court order. Mom approached Dad with the question that if things would go wrong, what would he want the staff to do? Dad answered that he didn't want a ventilator. I myself didn't want to think about the possibility that he might need one. I was unable to participate when Mom and Dean discussed it with the doctor.

When we met with the lung doctor, Dad was doing better than anticipated. He had a strong will to live. Instead of being concerned about resuscitation, we considered bringing Dad back to our local hospital so he would be close to home. We also considered the nursing care facility beside Flower Hospital as an intermediate facility. If Dad could be treated with oral medication instead of IVs, he would no longer be able to stay at the hospital. He had been a patient for nearly two weeks, and not much more could be done for him.

As Milan had done, Dean took the reins during the week he was in Ohio. I was relieved that both of them could spend quality time with Dad. The possible passing on of a father creates a need to reevaluate life's goals and think about one's own mortality.

Dean was especially concerned that Mom and I were not facing Dad's critical condition and were remaining too hopeful. Dean wanted us to consider cemetery plots and funeral arrangements. I tried to explain that being hopeful was how we had survived the past few months. Dean was impressed with how we had handled the situation, but now he said it was time to shift gears. I hated to think that Dad had endured the series of treatments in order to have this kind of existence. Yet, I would keep going as long as he wanted to fight. Each day was a precious gift, and the events are etched in my memory.

During these difficult days, two of my friends were particularly helpful. Renee had assumed my teaching duties with aplomb. It had been hard to stop teaching, and then be concerned about how things were going for a sub. Renee handled the classes well, and she thought of additional ways to assist me. She knew how she would feel if it was her father. She used her superb culinary skills to prepare meals for us. Upon our return from the hospital, we would find a full-course dinner on Mom's kitchen table. So, Renee was teaching, grading papers, and finding time to cook. Her generosity was truly appreciated.

Another good friend, Kayta, would call to ask about my day at the hospital. She knew the art of listening and not asking too many questions or becoming bored with repetition. She had her own busy schedule, yet she took time to show empathy.

Rev. Flinchbaugh met both my brothers and visited Dad from

time to time. When he asked Dad how he was doing, Dad answered that there had been times when he had felt better. Rev. Flinchbaugh told us that Dad had a healthy, mature personality inside a sick body. On occasion, Rev. Flinchbaugh joined us for lunch in the cafeteria, and we enjoyed his company.

While Dad was still in ICU, an impartial doctor, appointed by the Industrial Commission of Ohio, examined Dad and his medical records. He was not one of Dad's regular doctors, but the examination was one of the steps for the workman's compensation suit. The exam took place nine days after Dad had been admitted to the hospital.

In the doctor's report, the opening statement was, "The claimant is critically ill at this time, and is troubled with significant shortness of breath, but is oriented as to time and place, and the history, in my opinion, appears to be reliable." From his interview, the doctor wrote about Dad's recent cancer diagnosis and his work in the core room of the foundry. He wrote about Dad's past medical history, his health habits, and a review of his current symptoms. He then did his own physical examination, and looked over Dad's extensive medical records and tests. His summary and impressions are as follows:

Laboratory Studies:

Review of the records reveals that the claimant worked in Central Foundry in Defiance from 1950 to 1981. There was exposure to asbestos, according to the records. The claimant stated that he worked in the Core Department at the Central Foundry, and this department made and processed cores, rough castings for engine blocks. Furthermore, he states that the core room was extremely dusty. The overhead pipes were insulated with asbestos. The insulators worked 20 to 30 feet away during construction. The use of respirators was not enforced.

There is substantiation of a diagnosis of mesothelioma with the record revealing that a biopsy of the pleura revealed malignant tumors showing variable differentiation with ultra structural features, characteristic of mesothelioma (Diagnostic Specialty Laboratory, Bremerton, Washington).

Summary:

This 72-year-old gentleman has a history of well-documented mesothelioma, dating back to June of 1989. The claimant was treated with radiation therapy and chemotherapy, off and on since, and is now hospitalized at Flower Memorial Hospital in Sylvania, Ohio, in a terminal status with significant respiratory distress. On physical examination, the claimant appears acutely and chronically ill, and at least five years older than his stated age. He is tachypneic and is fibrillating with a rapid ventricular response. There is no neck distension. Examination of the chest reveals diminished to absent breath sounds of the right chest with a pleural friction rub on the right, and rales in the left chest posteriorly. Heart sounds are quite distant. The rhythm is irregularly irregular at 135 per minute. There is no murmur, however, rub, nor gallop. Examination of the abdomen is not remarkable. There is no clubbing and no cyanosis of the nailbeds.

Diagnosis: #1. Mesothelioma of the right chest. #2. History of recent pneumonia.

In reply to your questions, I trust that the following information will be helpful to you, as to whether the mesothelioma is a direct and proximate result of the industrial accident. It has been stated that as many as 80% of mesotheliomas may be associated with asbestos exposure. (Speizer, F.E.: Environmental lung diseases, in Harrison's *Principals of Internal Medicine*, lith ed. New York, McGraw-Hill, 1987, 1070.) There is a history of 30 years of potential exposure to asbestos with the claimant's statement that he was employed in the foundry for this period of time. It is my opinion that there is a very strong likelihood of a relationship between industrial exposure to asbestos and this claimant's mesothelioma.

As to the claimant's present impairment due to this disease, there would be a 100% degree of impairment and the condition is permanent.

The above report was signed by the examining physician. Several of the dates had been incorrectly typed, and revisions had to be made until that part of the report was correct. The rest was accurate.

Chapter 27
Giving a Deposition

About this time, Dean asked Dad if he was still interested in doing a deposition. Typically, a deposition is done six months after filing a suit, to allow the asbestos companies to personally question the plaintiff. If the judge granted permission, the deposition would take place at the hospital. Mr. Contrada, who by now had formed his own firm called Contrada and Associates, secured permission for the deposition. He served notices to the lawyers of companies named in the suit. Dad was very much in favor of doing the discovery deposition.

The hospital allowed the deposition only if Dad was moved to a room on the regular coronary floor. The size and comfort of his new room, across from the nurses' station, were pleasant changes. Dad received fewer IVs, and he took his medication orally. He still had an oxygen tube in his nose. Because his lungs were filling with fluid, he again received pulmonary machine treatments.

The day before the deposition, on a Sunday, Dad sat in the chair beside his bed and ate dinner. It was the first time he had been upright in two weeks, and Dad was full of determination. I began to think more positively. Dean had said Dad would get a little worse each day. Instead, Dad seemed to be improving. I began to hope for a full year, and maybe a longer survival. We talked with the doctor about moving Dad to Lake Park Nursing Care Center where the same doctors could care for him. We spoke of the move as a possible step forward in Dad's condition.

The deposition was scheduled for a Monday morning. Over the weekend, I worried. I didn't want the lawyers to embarrass Dad because of his critical condition. I knew how badly he wanted to do it, yet I didn't want him to overtax himself. Also, my witnessing the deposition might be too emotional.

On the morning of the deposition, Mr. Contrada met with the lawyers in a conference room by the nurses' station. Nine lawyers, representing various defendants, had come. Mr. Contrada advised them about Dad's current health condition and asked that the questions not be lengthy. He said that if there were objections, that one objection be made for everyone. Except for objecting to the form of the question or response, he asked that substantive objections be saved for the trial.

One lawyer claimed his corporation had not received notice about the deposition. Another lawyer asked if Mr. Grove had reviewed the picture book of asbestos products. Mr. Contrada said that Dad was not going to identify products, since that had been done by co-workers, witnesses, and persons who did insulation of pipe coverings.

One lawyer adamantly objected to the deposition, even though the suit had been filed nearly two months prior. He said he was not adequately prepared. He also said that the plaintiff's medical condition would prevent a complete inquiry into his work history.

In response, Mr. Contrada said that the doctors had agreed that Mr. Grove was capable of going forward with the deposition. He added that Dad's work history was very straightforward. In fact, the asbestos lawyers had been provided with a written consolidated discovery response months ago. After further discussion, Mr. Contrada stated, "Well, I think we'll be able to question him in a few minutes and see how the record develops."

The discovery deposition started as soon as Dad was officially sworn in. Mom sat at Dad's bedside, and Mr. Contrada sat on the opposite side. Lawyers stood about the room, and the court reporter and video cameraman stationed themselves near the foot of Dad's bed. Dean and I stood near the doorway. The first lawyer, smartly dressed in a suit, stood politely beside Dad as she questioned him. Dad stated his family history and UAW affiliation. Then she continued her questions to him:

Q. Mr. Grove, did you ever serve in the military?
A. No, ma'am.
Q. Have you ever smoked?
A. No.
Q. Mr. Grove, I understand that your first occupation was as a farmer, is that correct?
A. Yes, it was.
Q. Okay, and do you remember how old you were when you started farming?
A. Well, around 17.
Q. Seventeen. Did you work on your father's farm?

A. Yes, I did.

Q. Mr. Grove, what type of farming was it? Did you raise crops?

A. General farming.

Q. Okay, did you raise any livestock of any kind?

A. Oh, yes.

Q. Okay. What kind of animals did you have on the farm?

A. Hogs, cattle, chickens, and sometimes sheep.

Q. Do you remember using any fertilizers?

A. We didn't use it much in those days.

Q. What about pesticides?

A. We didn't use it.

Q. Did you ever work on farm machinery?

A. Yes. Yes, I repaired it.

Q. Did you ever replace any brakes on any of the machinery?

A. No. It didn't have much brakes on it.

Q. Did you ever replace brakes on cars and trucks?

A. No — not that I recall.

Q. Okay. Was it after farming that you began working at General Motors?

A. Yes, it was.

Q. Okay, and what year did you begin working at G.M.?

A. I hired in June 21st, 1950.

Q. Okay, and what division of G.M. were you at?

A. I was in the core room. They called it the core room.

Q. The core room?

A. Yes, ma'am.

Q. And I believe, Mr. Grove, according to some discovery responses, that this was at the foundry at Defiance, is that right?

A. Yes. Yes.

Q. Okay.

A. Defiance, Ohio.

Q. When did you retire?

A. January the 1st, 1981, officially.

Q. Okay. What did you do in the core room when you first started at G.M.?

A. I was a dryer changer.

Q. Dryer changer?

A. Yes.

Q. What did you have to do as a dryer changer?

A. Take metal dryers off of one rack or car and put them on another or — or just take them off for a while. They made different shapes of cores.

Q. Okay. What is it that is made at the foundry in Defiance?
A. What's that?
Q. What part of the car is made at the foundry in Defiance?
A. Gray iron parts.
Q. Okay. Over the thirty years that you worked there, did you have different job functions, or did you eventually have one?
A. No. I had different ones sometimes.
Q. Can you tell me what job functions you had?
A. Well, like making cores and relief man. A relief man works all over.
Q. Okay. Any other job functions that you remember?
A. Well, that was the main part of it.
Q. Okay, so as a relief man, you would have been all over the plant then?
A. No, just my area mostly.
Q. Okay. What—what area was that?
A. Well, that'd be around where we made the castings for the Oldsmobile and like that.
Q. During the time you were at the foundry, was there ever any remodeling of the plant?
A. Oh, yes.
Q. Do you remember approximately how many times you remember remodeling going on?
A. Well, about every winter they would start tearing the side blocks away and put — put up a plastic and start working away from us. They put up — they wrapped pipes with asbestos and as they moved away from us, it was dusty all over.
Q. Okay. So when they would wrap the pipe with asbestos —
A. That's what?
Q. When they would wrap the pipe with asbestos, they would put plastic up?
A. Yes, and move out of the way from you and keep building.
Q. Okay, so do you remember seeing insulators at the G.M. Foundry?
A. Yes.
Q. Do you remember any of the insulating contractors that may have been there?
A. I didn't personally know them.
Q. Okay. Other than wrapping that these insulators would put on pipe when the remodeling was going on, do you remember any other products which you believed contained asbes-

tos that would have been present?

A. Well, I didn't pay any attention because I didn't realize how dangerous it was.

Q. So are you able to identify for us today any names of products or manufacturers of products which were used at the G.M. Foundry —

A. Well —

Q. — that you believed contained asbestos?

A. Johns-Man-Manville, but they've gone bankrupt.

Q. Okay, but you remember seeing Johns-Manville products?

A. Yes.

Q. Do you remember what types of products you remember seeing that were made by Johns-Manville?

A. Well, mostly wrappings.

Q. Anything else that you can recall?

A. Not at the present.

Q. Okay, so is Johns-Manville the only product name or manufacturer name that you can remember as today?

A. Yes, as a regular name.

Q. Mr. Grove, do you remember when you worked at G.M. Foundry, if there were any chemicals or gases that you would have been exposed to?

A. Chemicals?

Q. Did you ever work with chemicals?

A. No — not in particular.

Q. What about any gases?

A. No, not really.

Q. Did you ever wear a mask or respirator when you worked at the G.M. Foundry?

A. Toward the last I did some.

Q. When you say "toward the last," do you mean like in the last ten years that you worked?

A. Yes.

Q. And when would you wear that mask?

A. Oh, usually when it was the dustiest. There were times when it was dustier than others.

Q. Okay. Mr. Grove, have any doctors told you that your present illness is related to asbestos exposure?

A. Yes, they have.

Q. And what doctors told you that?

A. Dr. _____ in Seattle, Washington. He was at the head of the cancer department.

The second questioner asked Dad if he felt up to continuing the questions, and Dad responded that he did. I was surprised at Dad's calmness. I thought he was doing very well. The second questioner sat on the floor at the foot of Dad's bed. Dad couldn't even see his face. The lawyer fumbled with a notebook in his lap. His first questions were about whether or not Dad wore any protective clothing at work. Then, he asked about the core room itself.

Q. How much time did you spend making up molds of cores — I'm sorry, cores?

A. Making cores?

Q. Yeah. I'm trying to get a feel for whether you spent most of your career making up cores or just a small part of your career making up cores.

A. I spent most of my career in — well, you could call in general labor. I made cores and was a relief man sometimes.

Q. Could you tell me how you'd go about making up a core?

A. Well, they had machines in the core room. Toward the last, they had an overhead system where they would drop their sand down chutes, just plain lake sand or silica sand, and the machines there, they were run by air. They would compress the sand into the shape and — of your dryers, you know.

Q. Can you explain what a dryer is?

A. A dryer is a piece of metal that holds your sand in the shape you want to dry it in.

Q. And then when the —

A. There's various sizes.

Q. All right, and let me see if I understand. Then, when the sand is dry, you can remove the metal dryer, and then you have a core, is that right?

A. Right.

Q. Okay.

A. That's solid enough to handle so that the metal won't penetrate for a little bit.

Q. Okay. What did you use to hold that sand together inside the metal dryer?

A. Well, the sand had a formula. It had what they call core oil and kerosene and several things that once you got that consistency right and it dried a little bit in there, it stayed in that shape.

Q. Would you be the person that was responsible for mixing

the sand and oils, or were they premixed? How did they come to you?

A. There were regular sand mixers that were experienced. I didn't do it very often. I have on occasion.

Q. When you'd be mixing sand for the cores, would that be one of the times that you'd wear a mask or not?

A. Well, they — they might have in later days. We didn't in the early days.

Q. Okay. What was the — the dustiest or dirtiest part of your job?

A. Well, it was dusty all over, but be hard — be hard to say.

Q. Just dusty all over, is that the idea?

A. Yeah.

Q. And when you say "all over," do you mean inside the foundry?

A. Yeah, swift — swift dust blowing all the time.

Q. Other than the sand and the oils and the metal dryers, were there any other products that you used in the foundry?

A. Well, there was a — what they call a dip. They had a dip room, and they would mix different consistencies together so they could — well, they could dip their cores in this. Now, you dipped a core out in the core room for the purpose of keeping metal from penetrating it for a little bit. You put water solution, sort of a covering, a dip on it or a paint you could call it.

Q. And you did that by actually placing the core in a bath of this liquid, is that the idea?

A. Right. Right.

Q. Do you know what was in that liquid or what it was composed of?

A. No, not really, unless you'd read on the sack real good. No, I don't know.

Q. Dipping the core in this liquid, was that part of your job?

A. Part of the time.

Q. Can you think of any other products or materials that you used throughout your career in the foundry?

A. No, not in relation to that.

Dad did fine at first. The deposition was lasting over an hour. The only inaccurate response was the size of the original foundry, which Dad could not remember. I think he gave the present square footage of the three plants instead of the width of the original plant. Dad did describe the number of employees and how automation reduced the number of employees over the years. He also described the frequent expansions and renovations which took place during the late fifties, the sixties, and the early seventies. I was proud of him.

After a short break following the discovery deposition, the videotaped deposition took place. I had thought the whole procedure would take fifteen to twenty minutes. Instead, Dad was beginning his second hour of testimony.

During the second hour, Mr. Contrada, our attorney, directly examined Dad. Dad answered questions about his personal life and family. He then told how the disease mesothelioma had affected his life, including the things he was no longer able to do. He again described his dusty work situation and the lack of protective apparel. Mr. Contrada was the questioner.

Q. You've discussed your surgery. Where was your surgery performed, Mr. Grove?

A. At the Swedish Hospital in Seattle, Washington.

Q. Why did you go to Seattle for your surgery?

A. Well, I had a son there that was a doctor and — he knows pretty much the ins and outs.

Q. Did you have any lung problems before all this with your — this illness that you're involved with?

A. Not until they diagnosed it as — as cancer.

Q. How was your health before they diagnosed the cancer?

A. Well, I thought it was excellent. I could — I could jog and run the treadmill and everything.

Q. Have you been able to do that since the cancer?

A. No. No. I can't — I can hardly breathe.

Q. During the 30 years at the General Motors Foundry, how many sick days would you have taken?

A. Probably not over ten.

Q. Between 1980 and when you had your cancer last year, did you go anywhere with your wife?

A. Well, we went to the commencement, the high school commencement at Bellevue, Washington.

Q. Would that be for your grandchildren?

A. Yes, we went to that, but —

Q. Other than Washington state, have you visited any other states of the union?

A. All of them.

Q. Have you ever visited outside the United States?

A. Yes.

Q. Where would that be?

A. Germany, Austria, and even Egypt and Greece and the Holy Land and the — the Iron Curtain States. Yeah. We've been in a lot of countries.

Q. What was the most enjoyable thing you did with your wife after retirement?

A. Well, I guess just general trips and things like that.

Q. Did you have to postpone any trips because of the cancer?

A. Well, I went on a little trip down to Nashville after I had cancer, but it wasn't very good. I got so I couldn't walk and get air, you know. I got worse.

Q. Did you have any treatment after your surgery last summer?

A. Yes, I had — at first, I had radiation every day for 41 days, plus every Tuesday, I had chemotherapy with it, but it got to the place where there were side effects, you know, that I couldn't take it any longer.

Q. What's the worst part of the illness that you have?

A. Well, I suppose not knowing whether I'll get over it or not, because it's — it's hard to fight this kind.

Q. Have you discussed the nature of your illness with your wife and children?

A. Well, yes, yes. They've been very close.

Q. Can you tell us a little bit about what you've discussed?

A. Well, they're very concerned about me and do everything they can for me, but we haven't — we discussed a little bit the odds of getting well, you know, for several years, but we don't know.

Q. Since you've been told about your illness, have you noticed any change in the way that your friends or family —

A. Oh, yes.

Q. — have related? How is that?

A. They've been much closer, from one end of the country to the other.

Q. Has anyone told you whether or not there's any real cure for the cancer that you have?

A. No, they haven't.

One of the lawyers objected to the testimony about the disease. He said he objected because Dad wasn't an expert on the disease of mesothelioma. Of course, Dad had been living with the daily reality of the disease for nine months. It had been confirmed by doctors and laboratory tests. We had also been researching the disease, yet the lawyer raised the objection that my father could not describe the disease adequately. Mr. Contrada rephrased the question.

Q. Let me ask you one other question, Mr. Grove. What is your understanding of the cancer that you have?
A. Well, they told me that it isn't — it isn't really considered curable.

There were more questions by the asbestos company lawyers about Dad's work at the foundry and his early work on the farm. They also asked about gases he had been exposed to at the foundry. They asked if he had ever worked in maintenance or in pouring metal. They also inquired about Dad's work in reroofing my parents' home. The last question was about working near or installing large furnaces in which Dad said he had never been involved.

As a final gesture, Dad had to waive the right to reread or review the deposition. The only changes could be typographical errors. This was standard procedure before the written document became final.

Afterwards, the court reporter remarked to me how well Dad had done during the deposition. We concluded that he had been less nervous than persons who are not in the extenuating circumstances of hospitalization.

Testimony had lasted over two hours. We were mentally and emotionally exhausted. We gave Dad a chance to rest. It was time to take Dean to the airport for his return to Seattle. He planned to bring his entire family to Ohio in just eleven days, during their spring break. After his move from CCU, Dad had already talked to all his grandsons on the phone.

I hated for Dean to leave, but I was reassured by the fact that he would return soon and that Dad might be strong enough to make the move to the nursing care center beside the hospital. Mom and I bid Dean good-bye. I presented him with a copy of Kevin Leman's book, *First Born*, which describes common characteristics of the oldest child. I often teased him about still "bossing" me. We would keep in touch until he returned.

Chapter 28
Saying Good-bye

For two days after the deposition, Dad slept most of the time. By the third day, he was more alert and talked with visitors, including my aunt and uncle. The same day, his chemotherapist came by the room. We already knew what had happened to Dad's heart and right lung. We didn't know whether or not anyone had thoroughly explained it to Dad. The doctor proceeded to describe Dad's internal condition to him. I wasn't present, but I can imagine Dad reacting to the news with careful consideration. I guess the doctor was giving Dad permission to let go, if he was ready.

During this time, Dad began telling us about his visions. It was as if he was already approaching another plane of existence. Even though Dad was groggy and confused, he vividly described the visions when we arrived and repeated them before we left. Dad was no longer very concerned about earthly things. As he lay in his hospital bed, he had time to think about his beliefs and what the afterlife would be like. Since death is also a psychological and spiritual process, he had certain questions which concerned him.

After his first night in intensive care, he had shared some of his regrets with our minister. If death was pending, he regretted leaving his family. He regretted being unable to finish his second term as church treasurer. And he regretted being unable to live long enough to see his great-grandchildren. I had not known about Dad's conversation with her until I spoke with her three weeks later about Dad's visions.

First, Dad said that Jesus and his mother, Mary, had appeared to him. I had a friend tell me that his sister had this vision shortly before she died. It didn't seem like an omen for survival. Regarding Dad's concern about whether or not there would be room for all religions in heaven, Dad received the answer that "we would all see the light of day." He added that it wouldn't matter what earthly creed or religion one had, Dad felt that his spiritual being would be ongoing on another plane of existence.

It sounded ecumenical to me. Since our denomination doesn't emphasize Mary as an intermediary between ourselves and God, I was surprised Dad mentioned her presence. And, that he endorsed all religions, or perhaps no one religion, puzzled me.

Dad also seemed to receive messages about how the second coming would take place. Since he assumed we all knew about the messages, he was concerned that we didn't understand. He marveled that God would be able to carry out His plans. Dad said that ages of information had been shown to him in just a few minutes on a screen. In fact, he implied that time was a man-made thing. Dad contented himself with these revelations. The one which struck me the most was that Dad referred to his great-grandchildren as if he had already met them or knew their spirits. Knowledge of them would represent Dad's future immortality.

In words, I am not doing justice to the depth of Dad's feelings as he conveyed these thoughts. I knew they were beyond my understanding, and yes, I considered Dad's current state of mind. Perhaps the visions were a special gift from God to a man who had endured much physical suffering in his last months. I could not question their authenticity because of my limited perceptions. I wished I could see them, too.

During a spring season of unpredictable weather, it had been a stormy Saturday. Dad was so tired, he spoke to us with his eyes closed. The director of social services came to discuss moving Dad to the nursing facility in two days. Since there was a covered walkway between buildings, it wouldn't be necessary for Dad to go outdoors. The director had arranged the move, and all we needed to do was sign papers at the front desk of the center. We didn't ask for Dad's input about the move.

It was March 10, which happened to be Dean's birthday. Dad kept asking us what the date was. Dad gave me a list of chores, and he reminded me to get certain parts checked on my car. Parents are forever parents, I thought. Dad had also been giving us a lesson in facing death. He seemed to be past his physical suffering, as if his chest pain was not as great of a concern. He politely let the nurses take care of his medical needs. He really seemed at peace. That afternoon, he said that he guessed it wasn't such a feat to live to be a hundred years old. He said that we would be separated, but it wouldn't seem like such a long time apart. I considered what Bernie Siegel had said — "that dying can be a healing, for someone who is tired, in pain, and in need of a rest."

Because of threatening weather, we left the hospital earlier than

usual, and bid Dad good-bye. He said that the nights were sometimes long. As we departed, Mom and I promised that we would
see him tomorrow. We said we loved him. "Same here," he had
replied.

The next morning I was to play the organ for church, and we
planned to leave after the service for the hospital. I had wanted to
rise early, but I couldn't seem to shake my lack of energy. In fact,
it felt as if some force was preventing me from opening my eyes.
When I did get up, the first thing I did was set my watch. It was
9:12 A.M. As I was fixing a cup of coffee, the phone rang.

Mom said a doctor from the hospital had called, and Dad was
having trouble. They had asked if they should continue CPR, and
Mom had told them not to. She asked me to get ready to go to the
hospital immediately. But, I thought, if the situation is that bad, I
don't want to witness it.

I called our minister to tell her I couldn't play for the service. I
said that Dad probably wouldn't make it through the day. My
mother phoned Dean, and she had him call the hospital. He called
her back to say that Dad had died at 9:12 A.M. At church, the minister turned on recorded music in the sanctuary, and then she
drove to my mother's house. That left no minister or organist,
which confused the congregation. Mom called both of my brothers
and then called me back. I asked if Dad had died, and she couldn't
get the words out. Finally, she just said, "Yes." I was numb. His
battle was over. It didn't seem real.

Like a trooper, Dad had eaten his breakfast that morning. Since
patients often die during the long night, I knew Dad had still been
fighting. I also knew that he had not wanted to die on my brother's birthday, the day before. I was aware that Dad was not particularly thrilled about going to a nursing home. Dad had fought
until the end, but his body had not cooperated. "What's a fellow to
do when his body doesn't do what it's supposed to?" he had
asked just a couple weeks earlier.

Before Dean's recent departure, Mom had asked him what he
wanted for his birthday. He had tearfully answered that he wanted
Dad to be free from his suffering. Dean had gotten his wish. Death
isn't the worst thing that can happen, I thought. The worst part
had been watching a loved one suffer, and not being able to do
something about it.

My uncle and aunt drove us to the hospital. I thought our pur-
pose was to sign the release papers. When the elevator arrived on
Dad's floor, Rev. Flinchbaugh was waiting for us. He embraced
Mom, and it was the first time I had seen her cry that day. The

nurses had thoughtfully contacted Rev. Flinchbaugh and told him we were coming. He explained that it was customary to leave the body in the room, so the family could spend time there, and the attending nurse could explain the circumstances.

When we entered the room, it seemed unusual that Dad didn't warmly greet us. It also seemed odd that his chest was still, and he was no longer struggling for breath. A blanket was folded around him. The nurse had packed his personal belongings in sacks. She had found Dad breathless after breakfast. CPR had been administered until code status was changed after contacting us.

Mom signed some release papers, as well as permission for a limited autopsy of the chest area. We informed the hospital personnel about which mortuary to contact. As soon as we left, the autopsy would be done at Medical College Hospital, another location in Toledo. After the autopsy was completed, the mortuary would transport the body to Bryan.

When the nurse left, we gathered around Dad, as we had done so often in recent weeks. We held hands while Rev. Flinchbaugh prayed. During the prayer, I placed my hand over Dad's to include him. I don't remember anything more we talked about.

My brothers' families planned to come at the end of the week. Our appointment with the funeral director was the next day. The minister and my uncle came to assist. The funeral director was very easygoing, but Mom still had trouble making simple decisions. We scheduled the funeral for Friday, so we had more time. We discussed ideas for the funeral and persons to contact. I wished my brothers could arrive sooner.

For the funeral folder, I decided to write a poem, to make it more personal. The poem was later read, at Dad's funeral. My poem is as follows:

Dad, we love you.
You were always there for us
in your quiet, dependable way.

And in your steady manner,
you lovingly guided us
and gave us opportunity for success.

We remember your legacy
of kindness, patience, concern,
of insight, discipline, and curiosity.

Even in your final challenge,
you taught us hope and courage
and that a loving Father
will gather His children home.

We know that you were the wisdom
and the quiet strength
lighting our journey.

Dad, we love you and thank you.

There were other decisions to make. We selected a wooden oak casket with a sculpture of the Lord's Supper on the side. It exemplified Dad's carpentry skills and his religious faith. We wanted flowers designated from the grandchildren, children, and wife. We also decided to have Dad hold a Bible with four roses to signify his four grandsons. We bought a section of plots at the cemetery where Mom's parents are buried.

That evening, members of my parents' Sunday School class came by the house. They came to offer support, to visit, and to reminisce. They were very loving. During the evening, I got some old photos out of a drawer and passed them around.

I wanted Dad's funeral to be a memorial tribute. We wanted several persons to speak, representing different aspects of Dad's life. Bill and Miriam Cable could speak as lifelong friends. Rev. Leland Grove, Dad's first cousin, could represent the family. And Paul Troder could speak as a fellow church member. Unfortunately, at first, none of these persons could be contacted. Even the organist was out of town. However, the soloist, Connie Gamble, a distant cousin, agreed to share her beautiful soprano voice. Since it was near Easter, we asked her to sing, "I Know That My Redeemer Liveth" from Handel's Messiah.

Our minister met with us as we chose scriptures and hymns. A hymn on my mind in recent weeks had been "Make Me a Captive, Lord." When in the hospital chapel, I had selected it on the computerized organ. The second verse held significance for me, because of witnessing Dad's unsteady and elevated heart rate, which I felt the words of George Matheson aptly referred to.

My heart is faint and low
Till it a master find;
It has no spring of action sure —
It varies with the wind.

It cannot freely move
Till Thou hast wrought its chain;
Enslave it with Thy matchless love,
And deathless it shall reign.

After selecting other congregational hymns, I hunted through Dad's shelves for an appropriate Bible to use in the casket. I hadn't realized that he owned so many versions and translations. I picked out two, and returned to the living room. Holding the Bibles behind my back, I exclaimed that I had found the perfect Bible to use — one that Dad could really enjoy. I whipped out the white carton of audio tapes called The Bible. Since Dad had a fairly new recorder and earphones, I suggested that those be included, too. My comments produced some light moments, as we all burst out laughing. Then, I showed them the Bible I had really chosen. Even Dad would have appreciated our sense of humor at that moment.

Contacting funeral participants was not an easy task. We finally located Bill and Miriam Cable in California, and they drove straight home to participate in the memorial service. Leland Grove was interrupted at a pastors' retreat, and he drove with his wife from Sioux City, Iowa, to Ohio. My cousin postponed a business trip to Europe in order to be a casket bearer. By the end of the week, plans for a meaningful memorial service had fallen into place. I arranged a display of family pictures to be shown at the funeral home. We decided that the memorial donations could be designated for the church.

Hundreds of persons came to the funeral home. One of the positive sides of funerals is the renewed relationships and friendships. Each visitor was truly appreciated. Two of my friends, who also had cancer, came. Persons who had worked with Dad, whom we had never met, came. One friend, who had not been inside a funeral home since her father's death fourteen years before, got up the courage to come. Colleagues and friends of my family members arrived. Even my sister-in-law's counselor from junior high camp reintroduced himself to her. We received numerous flowers and plants which were so beautifully arranged. Fortunately, the funeral director helps keep track of the kindnesses so that each person can later be thanked.

We especially appreciated persons who took time to write notes and letters to us. Following are excerpts from some of them.

I always wonder why such nice persons have to endure such unpleasant things. My only answer is that his courage was a living example that the problems I and others face on a day to day basis are not as major as we may think at the time. It also teaches us to enjoy the life that we have right here, right now. I will miss his friendly smile. He always made it such a pleasure to be in church since he took the time to greet my family and ask how we were doing. It was greatly appreciated.

Remember when:
   1. He helped with those CROP cardboard boxes and houses. He measured and cut doors and windows and helped put them together, roof and all.
   2. He made corn stalk wooden posts for corn shock table decorations at the retired teachers' meeting.
   3. He made little bird cages and hung them on a clothesline for the Apple Festival.
   Without him, we would have had to give up certain aspects of the projects that helped make each event a successful venture.

Kedric was a warm and charming man, and I am sorry for your loss.

I feel my life has been enriched by having known Kedric. He was a good man.

We will all miss Kedric very much. Paul recalls working at G.M. when Kedric was still there. Paul remembers Kedric as such a hard worker. Kedric was a kind and gentle man who will be remembered by all.

When we think of Kedric and the sturdy, wholesome life he lived, we are again reminded of the frailties that can confront us all. We shall always remember him with a deep sense of warmth and appreciation.

He was surely a good man and a wonderful neighbor. We know he suffered a lot with his illness, but he never complained to us about it. He just trusted and had a great faith.

We will always keep our fond memories of him at those many ballgames we attended together. Wasn't that fun!

His life was certainly one that can always give you pride. He was a pillar of the church and a loving father for his family.

Your father was happiest of all in his wonderful family. You can find comfort in knowing that you made his life very satisfying. I know that your memories of him will bring you lasting comfort.

Your father was a good Christian man who is going to be missed by many. It's hard to give up a parent when you have had a good and loving relationship. Maybe we can share some of our hurts and help each other in our healing process.

Your father's death is such a great loss, not only for you and your family, but for our whole church. To me, Kedric was a main corner-stone of our church. I had come to love your father as a dear church friend. He was one of the most interesting and intelligent men I had ever met. His mind was so sharp and his concerns so genuine. I loved to talk with him. It really hurt to see him suffer.

We know of no one who has consistently been more gentle, under-standing, patient, caring, and tolerant than Kedric, even in pain.

Your husband and Dad was a fine person who left behind a wonder-ful legacy to all of you, as well as to the church and community. He will be greatly missed.

These and other wishes of comfort and support are what become so necessary and meaningful when coping with a loss. The words emphasize the unique beauty of an individual life that has touched others. It is a reminder that how one faces adversity during illness can become a legacy to those who are left.

I was also touched by a group of my teaching colleagues who purchased a memorial tree in honor of my father. The tree was planted and dedicated on our church grounds.

We received two Catholic Mass cards. This indicates that a Mass has been spoken in honor of the deceased. One of the services, which took place in Chicago, was sponsored by my brother's com-pany. The other Mass was held in Philadelphia, and it was a gift from Milan's sister-in-law and her husband.

I had thought the funeral would be more difficult to get through. I steeled myself against the emotional part and tried to think of the event as a service of praise for Dad's life. I was pleased that everyone we had invited was able to participate. We left the casket closed at the church, trying to eliminate emphasis on the body. Some funeral customs seem archaic to me and that is one. Our family was escorted out of the service last. The four grandsons, along with two cousins and two church friends, served as casket bearers.

The Cables gave a loving memorial tribute as they spoke about first meeting my parents, and our joint family activities through the years. Leland Grove told about Dad's fascination with family connections. Paul Troder, with his fun-loving humor, even shared some jokes about Dad. The minister read scripture from Isaiah 40. All these sentiments, along with the music, were very moving.

After the funeral, Dean's family stayed for an additional week.

There was much paperwork involving the will, estate, insurance, and medical bills. The March weather was unseasonably warm, and we went on some day trips to see relatives and friends. We were already missing my Dad's mechanical skills when neither the front nor the back screen doors would latch at my mother's house, and the plumbing backed up. At my house, the electrical power went out and the dishwasher spewed forth smoke. Where is a Dad when you need one?

One bit of advice I would give others is to clean out your drawers now. People are going to go through them when you're gone. Their contents become a source of information and fascination. Dad had some interesting old photographs of himself when he was young. He had also saved an album of drawings which he had done as a little boy. I wondered why I had never known about Dad's artistic ability. We found a porcelain crucifix in a box, which we decided to give my nephew Jared for his forthcoming confirmation in the church.

It is difficult to go through personal belongings of a loved one. Removing them is like admitting they are gone and closing the door. Dad's cane stood beside the bed, along with the weights he had used for exercising. I could still picture him straining to gain a little more strength. The end had come much sooner than we planned.

Mom did not sort through Dad's clothes for several weeks. There was really no hurry, and I told her to do it when she was ready. Since Dad had several good suits, Mom sized up men she thought were Dad's height. She was grateful that a man in our congregation could make use of them.

While Mom was cleaning out Dad's pockets, she discovered an amusing thing. Dad's pockets were filled with almost any item one might need. Of course, we knew that Dad usually set off alarms at airport securities because of the coins in his pockets. And we knew he always had many useful articles on hand. I sometimes thought he surely must wear heavy-duty belts just to hold up his trousers. But the day of revelation had come, and as Mom took his clothes from the closet, she found a wealth of materials. There were postage stamps, 17 pencils, 9 pens, 46 paper clips, a safety pin, a key, 8 tacks, 2 screws, 5 handkerchiefs, numerous toothpicks, several memorandums, a pair of gloves, a bookmark, 8 quarters, 22 dimes, 11 nickels, and 44 pennies. No wonder he could pack so lightly when he went on vacation. His pockets were already well-supplied.

I had been back in school for only two weeks when Mom called me. She said she had lost a lot of blood, and did I think she should call a doctor? Initially, after Dad's death, not going to the hospital every day had been like a release, a sudden vacation. Now, Mom was having symptoms which demanded immediate attention. She made a doctor's appointment. After meeting with him, he scheduled some preliminary tests. When the source of the bleeding could not be found, the doctor suggested that Mom be admitted to the local hospital for further tests. Perhaps Mom was not getting along as well as I thought. Or maybe her body was just now reacting to the strain of the past few months. What if it was something serious?

When we met with the doctor, he mentioned four or five potential problems Mom might have. The least serious was a burst blood vessel, and the most serious was colon cancer. He recommended further tests to investigate the problem. Mom spent four days in the hospital. After an evening of drinking Go-Lightly, she had a lower GI. We decided Go-Lightly was a misnomer. Her red blood cells were low. However, no source of bleeding was found, even after an upper GI a week later. Thank goodness the bleeding had stopped, and no further problem was discovered.

My brothers made additional visits to assist Mom. Dean had a medical meeting in Indianapolis, and then came to Ohio with his wife. They energetically cleaned Mom's attic and garage. We soon firmly believed that Dad had exercised his penchant for never throwing anything away. My aunt and uncle had already hauled away one load of items from the garage. Dean and Mary did a more thorough second cleaning.

Milan spent a weekend cleaning Dad's workroom in the basement. Dad had constructed many projects there. When he couldn't find a needed tool, he would go out and buy a new one. During Milan's cleanup operation, he found duplicates of many tools. I guess a truly creative person is so engrossed in his work, he can't be concerned about organizing his equipment!

Mom's neighbor, Mary, helped her in innumerable ways. Mary is skilled at many tasks and possesses a golden heart. The common phrase about being "a brother's keeper" could be rewritten as "a neighbor's keeper" to describe Mary. A mere thanks would be insufficient in praising Mary for her assistance and valuable friendship.

When my brothers left, they said that the next cleaning chore would be Dad's barn, and they appointed me for the task! I told Milan he had cleaned the basement by moving boxes to the barn. I suggested that we could schedule future weekends for their return to clean the barn. However, we're still negotiating the project!

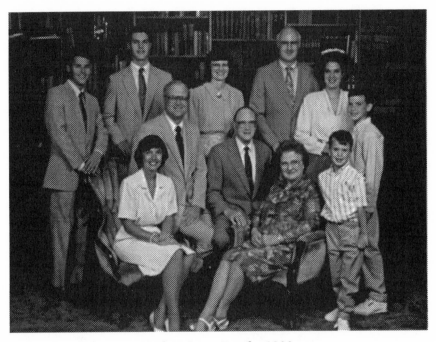

Kedric Grove Family, 1988

Chapter 29
Examining the Cancer

The official death certificate, issued by Lucas County, listed Dad's usual occupation as a core room worker in a foundry. The certifying physician wrote the immediate cause resulting in death as "malignant mesothelioma of the right lung" with approximate interval between the onset and death as nine months. The underlying cause which initiated events resulting in death was listed as "asbestosis." Another significant condition was "cardiac arrhythmia."

The autopsy was restricted to an examination of the chest and abdomen. The first part of the autopsy contained a synopsis of information from Dad's medical records during the past several months. The report, written by the Medical College of Ohio, was issued March 19, 1990, though we did not receive it for about two months.

The medical synopsis and correlation were as follows:

Kedric Grove was a 72-year-old man who died on March 11, 1990. This patient had worked at the Defiance General Motors Foundry from 1950 to 1981, retiring at the age of 63 years. During this 31 years of working at the General Motors Foundry, he had been allegedly exposed to asbestos. The patient had no history of smoking cigarettes.

During a routine physical examination by his physician in Bryan, Ohio, in the spring of 1989, an asymptomatic pulmonary nodule was discovered. A CAT scan of the chest, followed by needle biopsy of the lesion, revealed abnormal cells but no definitive diagnosis. A subsequent biopsy conclusively established the diagnosis of malignant neoplasm.

The patient moved to Washington state to undergo further treatment which included extensive decortication and resection of the neoplastic mass. The patient returned to Toledo where he had been actively followed in the Oncology Center at Flower Hospital for treatment of malignant mesothelioma. His treatment protocol included radiation therapy to the pleura followed by systemic chemotherapy with Adriamycin, administered every third week.

The patient was admitted to Flower Memorial Hospital on

January 11, 1990, with cough and right chest pain. Physical examination at that time revealed marked splinting of the right hemithorax on inspiration and reduced breath sounds throughout the entire chest. Coarse breath sounds were audible throughout the left lung base and crepitant rales were also heard. Chest X-rays at that time revealed extensive consolidation of the right lung with definitive infiltrates of the left lung. The impression at that time was probably pneumonia and/or atelectasis (collapsing) of the right lung.

On the 24th of January, a bronchoscopy was undertaken with the impression given of chronic inflammation and scarring of the right lung with mucus plugging and moderate generalized inflammation. Bronchial washing showed atypical cells. The patient was discharged on January 26, 1990, with visiting nurse support and instructions to follow-up in the clinic.

A few weeks later, the patient required readmission due to increasing shortness of breath. At this time, he was found to have atrial fibrillation and rapid ventricular rates as high as 180 per minute. On March 11, 1990, the patient was found breathless and in ventricular fibrillation. CPR was begun and continued until code status was changed as instructed by the family.

Upon examination of the chest and abdomen during autopsy, there was virtual fusion of the two layers of the right pleura by dense, fibrous adhesions.

Right lung

The right lung was a firm mass with a white-black appearance. Microscopic examination confirmed the presence of scattered foci of neoplasm, compatible with mesothelioma. The state of the lung was secondary to the presence of cancer and the attending therapeutic measures. The right lung showed no evidence of functional capacity. The trachea were occluded in many places with mucus plugging.

Left lung

The left lung was freely mobile in the chest. It was reddish-grey and the pleural surface was smooth and glistening. The left lung and pleural cavity were occupied by approximately 1500 ml of serous fluid. Considering this lung was the only functioning respiratory tissue, breathing would be severely compromised by this fluid. The resulting compromise would be considered a leading contributory factor in the cause of death.

A single fibrous adhesion on the anterior surface, along with a small visceral pleural nodule, was seen on the left lung. The hard nodule on the left upper lobe, which measured 1 cm, appeared to consist of a focus of neoplasm. There was a moderate to marked degree of anthracotic (dust) pigmentation outlining the pleural lymphatic system. Marked anthracotic pigmentation was seen in all sections of the lung.

Metastases of tumor

The bulk of the neoplasm (cancerous growth) appeared to reside in the right chest cavity, but had extended considerably into the mediastinum (middle of the thorax) occupying the pericardial sac (sac surrounding the heart) and surrounding the lower two thirds of the esophagus. The pericardial space was completely obliterated by fibrinous adhesions. It is likely that the tumors stimulated this condition. The inflammation of the sac around the heart was sufficient to have had some impairing impact on the functional capacity of the heart.

Heart

The heart chambers were of normal size, and there was a single nodule on the atrial surface. Malignant mesothelioma was scattered throughout the superficial layer of tissue around the heart. There was also dense, fibrous connective tissue. However, there was no evidence of infarction.

Appearance of tumor

Malignant neoplasm was present in all sections of the right lung. The tumor appeared to grow in streaming arrays, blending imperceptibly with fibrous reaction. The appearance of the tumor was largely sarcomatoid in type, having a fairly abundant desmoplastic diffuse accompanying reaction. Numerous areas of necrosis (death of tissue) and hemorrhage were seen throughout sections of the right lung.

Liver

Fibrous strands were also seen infiltrating the liver. Two focal nodules on the right lateral lobe of the liver were noted on the external surface. These hard nodules were pearl-white and extended into the liver.

Location and description of tumor

The tumors around the right lung and pericardial sac were the main focus of the neoplasm. In addition, the small nodule on the left pleura and two metastatic nodules in the liver comprised the rest of the visible neoplasm. The neoplasm itself was composed principally of spindle type cells, although vaguely epithelioid forms could be seen as well. Particularly in the lung, but also in the pericardium, there was an accompanying desmoplastic reaction. This appearance corresponded to the so-called sarcomatoid type of mesothelioma.

It's a revelation to find out what conditions a cancer patient has been fighting. Until the autopsy, there's no way of knowing for sure where the cancer has spread. On one hand, knowledge beforehand may have been too much to cope with. However, afterward, finding out is a confirmation that debilitating treatments were not unwarranted. One wonders how Dad survived as long as he did. And, considering the metastases of the disease, it is a relief that further suffering did not take place.

In a video program on asbestos-caused diseases, I viewed patients diagnosed with mesothelioma who were actually in worse condition than Dad had been. They were living skeletons. Such a future course would have become even more difficult to witness.

When Dad was first diagnosed, Dean gave me an article from a medical journal. A physician had written about his wife's rare form of cancer. Even though it hardly ever occurred, he prayed for his wife's cancer to metastasize to her brain. He knew this would cause a much quicker, less painful death. Soon afterwards, his prayer was granted and his wife died.

At the time, I wondered why my brother gave me such a story. It seemed like an unusually cruel outcome. Now, however, I understood. I know that my father's suffering, as bad as it was, would have become worse. He had a cancer nodule in his remaining lung as well as nodules in his liver. And the doctors had been right about the tumors surrounding his heart.

I wouldn't wish this cancer on anyone. Fighting a losing battle can be a strain. The lack of effective treatment and the rapid progression of the disease contribute to the stress. Even so, my father fought the disease with a valiant spirit, and he lived his last days in an uplifting way.

Would Dad have fared as well and suffered less without the treatments? That is a difficult question for which there is no answer. The need to learn about the disease and do something is great. Taking treatments helps one actively deal with the illness. One receives knowledge and sympathetic support from various health care professionals. In taking treatments, one knows he has tried to combat the cancer. As long as there is a glimmer of hope, it is worth reaching for. And if learning about the progression of the disease extends medical science, it is even more worthwhile.

My father did not pass on the legacy of giving up. Life held much joy and fascination for him. In even the grimmest circumstances, he chose life. He did not do this because he feared death or belittled the afterlife. He just felt being alive was a precious gift.

Chapter 30
Environmentally-Caused Cancer

Asbestos is only one of many recognized hazardous materials our society has used or continues to use. The delay in dealing with asbestos and its disease potential has been an example for our industries and environment. There is no evidence that there is a safe level of exposure for any carcinogen. However, OSHA has again proposed to lower the industry limits of asbestos from 2 fibers per cubic centimeter of air to .5 f/cc (Dreher, 1988, 229).

Currently, industries are studying substances in use. Industry is concerned that a substance in the workplace could be the next asbestos. More testing and gathering of information about a substance's safe use is being done beforehand (Rothstein, 1984, 187). The American Cancer Society has identified thirty agents used in industry which cause cancer. Most have been identified only after someone contracted disease. In addition, many more questionable materials in our environment have not been fully screened.

It is estimated that 70-90 percent of cancers are caused by environmental factors such as sunlight, X-rays, and radiation. Harmful chemicals cause 5-10 percent of cancers. Smoking, including secondary smoke, is also a leading cause of cancer (Johnson and Klein, 1988, 24-28). Health standards, which regulate toxic substances, require a series of medical procedures. An employer must conduct physical examinations beforehand and then conduct periodic exams. Citations and penalties can be issued for failure to do so (Rothstein, 1984, 19).

My goal has been to share what the common person can learn about the carcinogen, asbestos, and its diseases. I felt there was a need for general knowledge and a personal story, not just technical statistics. As my research developed into a larger puzzle, I wondered what our society has valued and why there has been such lack of awareness about the reality of asbestos-related disease.

My story is the experience of one man who tried to treat his asbestos-caused cancer, and found it impossible to stop its spread. While I can appreciate his many years of life as a parent of quality, I cannot be silent about his final struggle. His experience could happen to anyone. It is the reason we need to be educated about asbestos and its containment. Knowledge is the key to preventing further asbestos exposures and diseases. Hopefully, with this awareness, asbestos diseases will disappear after the next twenty years.

In listing what I learned from an experience in dealing with carcinogenic cancer, I include the following:

1. Cancer is a breakdown in the body's immune system. Such a breakdown can be caused by a carcinogenic agent.

2. Environmentally-caused cancer can occur in families with no prior history of cancer.

3. One can be around cancer-causing substances unknowingly.

4. There is usually a latent period between exposure and onset of disease.

5. Asbestos exposure really is dangerous and life-threatening.

6. The cancer can spread while there are no known physical symptoms outwardly apparent.

7. There is not a success rate for treating some kinds of cancer.

8. After the diagnosis, dealing with cancer becomes a way of life, since there is no remission period.

9. Doctors don't always have an answer nor are they able to detect where the cancer has spread.

10. Knowledge of the disease, and the support of family, friends, and healthcare professionals can be a lifeline.

Life goes on. Most of our legal cases were settled out of court. As medical bills came in, they were sent from one insurance company to another. Organized records are important, and we were fortunate to receive assistance from the insurance benefits director at the foundry. When illness confronts one member of a family, it confronts them all. Each suffers with the patient, and the family's need for support may not be as obvious. The grieving process continues for more than a year after the death. But, it is possible to work through the process and gain a renewed spirit and joy for living. From time to time, there are reminders of one's loss. But these can also remind one of his good fortune in having had a loving parent who, despite his final illness, lived a fulfilling life.

As I think of my father's final days, his life conveyed the words in Paul's second letter to Timothy:

> As for me, already my life is being poured on the altar, and the hour for my departure is upon me. I have run the great race, I have finished the course, I have kept the faith. And now the prize awaits me, the garland of righteousness which the Lord, the all-just Judge, will award me on that great Day; and it is not for me alone, but for all who have set their hearts on his coming appearance (II Timothy 4:6-8).

References

Agran, L. 1977. *The cancer connection and what we can do about it.* Boston: Houghton Mifflin Company.

American Cancer Society Statement. 1982. Public Issues Committee.

American Lung Association. *See* Asbestos.

Anderson, L. E., ed. 1990. *Mosby's medical, nursing, and allied health dictionary.* 3d ed. St. Louis: The C.V. Mosby Company.

Asbestos. 1986. American Lung Association.

Atchison, S.D. 1989. *Just when Manville thought it was safe.* Business Week, November 20, 36.

Barrett, J.C., P.W. Lamb, and R.W. Wiseman. 1989. *Multiple mechanisms for the carcinogenic effects of asbestos and other mineral fibers.* Environmental Health Perspectives 81: 81-89.

Boyle, R.H., and Environmental Defense Fund. 1979. *Malignant neglect.* New York: Alfred A. Knopf.

Bremner, B. 1989. *Asbestos makers run out of breathing room.* Business Week, November 20, 36-38.

Brodeur, P. 1985. *Outrageous misconduct.* New York: Pantheon Books.

Castleman, B.I. 1986. *Asbestos: medical and legal aspects.* Englewood Cliffs, N.J.: Prentice Hall Law and Business.

Cousins, N. 1989. *Head first: the biology of hope.* New York: E.P. Dutton.

Dreher, H. 1988. *Your defense against cancer: the complete guide to cancer prevention.* New York: Harper and Row.

Fletcher, D., M.D. 1988. *Asbestos: remove it? or leave it alone?* Medical Self-Care, Nov./Dec., 32.

Fulghum, R. 1989. *All I really need to know I learned in kindergarten.* New York: Villard Books.

Gilson, J.C. 1972. *Asbestos. Occupational health and safety.* Vol. 1. New York: McGraw-Hill Book Company.

Goldberg, M., M.D. 1988. *Cell wars: the immune system's newest weapons against cancer.* New York: Farrar, Straus, and Giroux, Inc.

185

Johnson, J., and L. Klein. 1988 *I can cope: staying healthy with cancer.* Minneapolis: DCI Publishing.

Johnson, L.P., M.D. 1989. *Pathology Report No. 88-M-15,* 253. Seattle: Laboratory of Pathology of Seattle, Inc.

Kohlberg, R. 1989. *Government issues final asbestos ban.* Washington, D.C.: United Press International.

Merchant, J.A., ed. 1986. *Occupational respiratory diseases.* Washington, D.C.: U.S. Department of Health and Human Services.

Merewether, E.R.A. 1930. *The occurrence of pulmonary fibrosis and other pulmonary affections in asbestos workers.* Journal of Industrial Hygiene 12: 198-222.

Mills, J., and E. Phillips, M.D. 1990. *Autopsy No. A-90-27.* Toledo: Medical College Hospital Department of Pathology.

Mossman, B.T., and J.B.L. Gee. 1989. *Asbestos-related diseases.* The New England Journal of Medicine 320:1721-1730.

Mossman, B.T., J. Bignon, M. Corn, A. Seaton, and J.B.L. Gee. 1990. *Asbestos: scientific developments and implications for public policy.* Science 247: 294-301.

National Cancer Institute Research Report. 1985. *Mesothelioma.* NCI Pub. 85-1847.

NCI Pub. 85-1847. *See* National Cancer Institute Research Report.

OEA. *See* Ohio Education Association.

Ohio Education Association. 1983. *Asbestos: is it a hazard in your school?* Ohio Schools, January 10-12, 20.

Peters, G.A., and B.J. Peters. 1980. *Sourcebook on asbestos diseases.* New York: Garland Press.

Pramik, M.J. 1985. *Bronchoscopy: a direct examination of your airways.* Krames Communications.

Robinson, P.M., ch. 1979. *Pastors' manual: Church of the Brethren.* Elgin, Illinois: The Brethren Press.

Rothstein, M.A. 1984. *Medical screening of workers.* Washington, The Bureau of National Affairs, Inc.

Sheler, J.L. 1987. *Asbestos: a back to school hazard.* U.S. News and World Report 103: 33.

Siegel, B.S., M.D. 1989. *Peace, love, and healing.* New York: Harper and Row.

Skinner, H.C.W., M. Ross, and C. Frondel. 1988. *Asbestos and other fibrous materials.* New York: Oxford University Press.

Sun, M. 1986. *EPA proposes ban on asbestos.* Science 231: 542-543.

Times-Post News Service. 1990. *Removing asbestos opposed.*

UMC. *See* United Methodist Communications.

United Methodist Communications (producer). 1984. *Growing through grief: personal healing.* Six videos. 30 min. each. Nashville: EcuFilm.

WBGH Television (producer). 1984. *Asbestos: a lethal legacy.* 57 min. Boston: Time-Life Video.

Whelan, E., M.D. 1978. *Preventing cancer: what you can do to cut your risks by up to 50 percent.* New York: W.W. Norton and Company, Inc.

Whitaker, L. 1989. *Monster in the closet.* Time 133: 53.

Winter, R. 1979. *Cancer-causing agents: a preventative guide.* New York: Crown Books.